Escaping the Voices: A Guide to Reversing Chronic Depression

EVAN HOWARD

Published by Pedigree, 2024.

While every precaution has been taken in the preparation of this book, the publisher assumes no responsibility for errors or omissions, or for damages resulting from the use of the information contained herein.

ESCAPING THE VOICES: A GUIDE TO REVERSING CHRONIC DEPRESSION

First edition. November 19, 2024.

Copyright © 2024 EVAN HOWARD.

ISBN: 979-8230843559

Written by EVAN HOWARD.

ESCAPING THE VOICES

A Guide to Reversing Chronic Depression

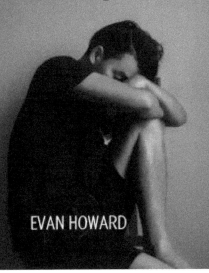

EVAN HOWARD

Table of Contents

INTRODUCTION 1
CHAPTER 1 | UNDERSTANDING THE DEPTHS OF CHRONIC DEPRESSION 4
   The Silent Weight of Persistent Sadness 7
   The Physical Toll of Mental Pain 10
CHAPTER 2 | IDENTIFYING AND CHALLENGING NEGATIVE THOUGHT PATTERNS 13
   The Cycle of Negative Self-Talk 17
   Rewriting Inner Narratives 21
CHAPTER 3 | NURTURING EMOTIONAL RESILIENCE AND SELF-COMPASSION 24
   Building Emotional Resilience in Everyday Life 28
   Practicing Self-Compassion and Kindness 31
CHAPTER 4 | HEALING THROUGH LIFESTYLE CHANGES AND DAILY ROUTINES 34
   The Role of Sleep and Nutrition 38
   Movement, Exercise, and Mental Health 42
CHAPTER 5 | BUILDING MEANINGFUL CONNECTIONS AND SUPPORT SYSTEMS 46
   Recognizing the Power of Community 50
   Asking for Help Without Fear 54
CHAPTER 6 | MINDFULNESS, MEDITATION, AND ALTERNATIVE THERAPIES 58
   The Benefits of Mindfulness in Daily Life 62
   Exploring Complementary Therapies 66
SUMMARY 70

INTRODUCTION

Thoughts circle like vultures when walls shut in. Every waking moment seems like a war, with darkness encroaching on the borders and an unseen weight on each breath. Many people experience despair in whispers, persistent, nagging voices that question every word, every look, and every opportunity for brightness. And as time passes, it becomes more difficult to determine if those murmurs are falsehoods or distorted realities that begin to conflate. It's a gradual suffocation that is concealed in little things like going to the shop, looking in the mirror, or acting normal among other people. How much longer can someone bear that burden before it becomes ingrained in their soul?

This is a battle with something deeper, something that settles within, something that resists all efforts to shrug it off, rather than a battle against grief. This isn't the kind of grief that goes away after a day off. Chronic depression lurks in the background, unexpectedly showing up during serene periods. It appears when you least expect it to, tainting the brightest days and creeping in when you thought you were at last free. It is unrelenting. It's clever. Additionally, it is well aware of which vulnerabilities to exploit and which fears to exacerbate. It waits patiently because it knows that when your defenses are down, it will reappear even if you ignore it for a day. That is this beast's nature.

But in the midst of all of this, a seed of rebellion sprouts, subtly retorting, opposing the voices, and fighting the darkness. And no matter how weak or little it may seem, that little resistance is what has potential. Beyond the years of heavy silence and under all the layers of self-doubt, there is a chance to begin resisting. Finding the patterns, following the channels of thought as they spiral, and understanding the traps the mind creates for itself are the first steps. One thread at a time, you begin to dismantle those patterns as soon as you can clearly see them. You begin to challenge, question, and reshape those voices until they are no longer powerful.

IT'S NOT A STRAIGHT line. It's chaotic, full of disappointments that make you feel like a failure and times when you think all of your effort may have been for nothing. However, even if it is small, progress seems like the slow warming that follows a hard winter. You also learn to recognize the deceptive tactics of sadness, including how it takes energy, messes with habits, and isolates with the subtlety of a slow poison. You begin looking for methods to recover these stolen parts, going back to healthy eating habits, sleep schedules, and other daily self-care activities that, while they may not seem like much, gradually develop a quiet resilience.

Fundamentally, recovering from persistent depression calls for a certain sort of fortitude that transcends common health and self-help recommendations. It requires introspection and a direct confrontation with the tales you've told yourself, the way your mind has been programmed, and the way you've lived through these cycles—often automatically. Real change starts in those candid moments, which are often unvarnished and perhaps unpleasant. It seems like tearing open wounds to peel back these layers, yet with each one gone, a brighter, more genuine glance shows through. It's a process of self-reclamation, a gradual but significant restoration of self-worth and confidence that had been buried behind years of suffering and uncertainty.

SIMPLE BUT DEEP TRUTHS become apparent as the cacophony of despair subsides, even if only momentarily. It demonstrates that the means of survival—movement, awareness, and deep connections—have always been accessible. These aren't fast fixes or miracle cures, but dependable allies along the journey, routines that shatter the stillness that sadness thrives in, and habits that turn into lifelines. It's difficult to develop these habits, particularly when sadness tells you there's no need. But every time you overcome that voice and go beyond that reluctance, it becomes less powerful.

Ultimately, this isn't about changing who you are or forgetting the past. It's about embracing the darkest parts of your narrative, integrating them all, and figuring out how to carry them without letting them consume you. Recovering from depression is a difficult and often frustrating process that involves rewriting the present with hard-earned realities and unlearning old narratives. Even though the shadows will always be there, you start to see them as a component of the scenery rather than the whole image.

The fragments of freedom are delicate at first, but they become stronger every time you confront the voices, get up, and go on with your day without being bound by the burden of a quiet struggle. You recover the life that has always been yours through every upswing, every descent, and every voice that wanes in the distance.

CHAPTER 1
UNDERSTANDING THE DEPTHS OF CHRONIC DEPRESSION

Even on the clearest days, dark, heavy clouds loom over the planet, and despite the noise of the outer world, a quiet soon follows. Like a continuous leak, chronic depression creeps in subtly until it permeates every aspect of life and establishes roots in the body, mind, and soul. It gets ingrained in your breathing, your morning greetings, and your way of moving through the world. It's more than simply melancholy or exhaustion; it's a landscape of perpetual weight that follows everywhere and casts shadows where hope once shone. Many people experience persistent sadness as the voice in the back of their minds that keeps raising questions and eroding their sense of value until every accomplishment and every effort at pleasure seems false. And in this perverted familiarity that makes the darkness seem like a natural part of you, the struggle starts in silently, without sirens or warnings.

Living beneath that shadow teaches you its language, including its falsehoods, whispers, and methods of persuading you that you are damaged and irrevocably different. Depression doesn't yell; instead, it steals happiness in quiet, inconspicuous moments, such as sitting with friends and feeling a fog in the distance, reaching out for connection only to experience a strange emptiness in return. Before it reaches the throat, laughing is silenced, vivid hues become gray, and everything it touches loses its shine, reducing the world to a monotonous muddle. Even the recollection of what it was like to live without this shadow wanes as the days start to blend together.

The endurance of persistent depression is what makes it so pernicious. One day you could push through it, and the following day you might discover it has come back. Without knowing the nature of the beast you're confronting, others around you may give counsel like "Just think positively" or "Get over it," which is supposed to ease temporary misery. A motivating statement or a night out won't solve this problem. Reprogramming reactions and altering mental patterns are two ways that chronic sadness permeates the very fabric of the mind. It's like having a voice that is completely capable of destroying any hope in a matter of seconds. It is always there, waiting to drag you back down, whenever you attempt to get up or recover even a little bit of pleasure.

THEN THERE IS THE BODILY burden, a limb heaviness, a deep aching that is difficult to describe in words. Sleep is both a haven and a prison, yet the fatigue doesn't go away even after spending hours in bed. A persistent and unyielding fatigue seeps into the bones. Every work gets more difficult than the previous, and energy becomes scarce until it seems impossible to get out of bed. Even while it demands interaction, life becomes more and more alone as it constricts within the confines of one's own thoughts. Like an imperceptible wall that becomes thicker every day, depression isolates a person in a manner that words cannot adequately describe, drawing them away from friends, family, and even from themselves.

Years pass, and the numbness becomes used to it—in a strange way, even consoling. After all, numbness indicates that you are experiencing something other than the unidentified sensation of loss and intense pain. But the greatest portions, the times that used to matter, are also taken away by numbness. Together with the negative, it dulls the positive until recollections of happiness and genuine laughing seem far away, as if you were seeing someone else's life on a screen. Depression rewires what it means to feel, to connect, and to hope the longer it persists. It makes you believe that this is the norm and that happiness is a fantasy that only exists for other people, not for you.

However, there is still a spark of resistance somewhere in all of this. Even while it may be quiet, a voice hardly audible above a whisper, it persists and pushes back in seemingly inconsequential ways, like choosing to get out of bed, even if just to sit by a window, or reaching out to someone when the want to talk becomes overwhelming. Little acts of rebellion that serve as a reminder that the darkness hasn't completely prevailed, even if they are subtle. Because depression cannot erase all of a person's resilience, no matter how strong it is. Every decision to continue, no matter how little, turns into a silent act of resistance and serves as a reminder that there is still a part of you struggling to live.

THERE ARE TIMES, HOWEVER fleeting ones, when this resistance intensifies and a glimmer of light breaks through the shadows. It's the choice to attempt, even if you have deep-seated concerns about its success. the choice to ask for assistance, to search for solutions in previously unconsidered areas, and to have the dim hope that life may have something more to offer than this shadow. Chronic depression doesn't go away quickly, but as you start to see the falsehoods it tells, a change and gradual unwinding may happen. Every step forward breaks the quiet a little more, but healing begins as a series of decisions, a journey that is full of detours and turns.

To escape this depth, one must be prepared to investigate the physical and emotional costs that are connected to mental health. Depression affects the body just as much as the intellect, often in ways that are invisible. A vicious loop that feeds the mental weight is created when the immune system deteriorates, stress hormones rise, and sleep cycles break down. Regaining health from many perspectives is made possible by realizing this relationship. One little, intentional decision at a time, learning to nurture the body with exercise, sleep, and food turns into a kind of self-care, a quiet reawakening of what it means to feel human again.

Allowing depression to take control is not the same as learning to live with it and comprehending its subtleties and patterns. Rather, it's a kind of silent, persistent strength that strengthens with time, becomes more resilient, and starts to see through the deceptions of despair. Every epiphany, every choice to go on, is a little triumph, a fragment of oneself recovered from the shadows. That regained self becomes stronger and more rebellious over time, even in the face of darkness, until the weight no longer seems so heavy. Because there is a will, a voice that endures, that won't go away, hidden behind the layers of uncertainty and quiet.

The Silent Weight of Persistent Sadness

Every thought and movement is infused with that dull agony that lies somewhere between the chest and the pit of the stomach, making every step seem like dragging through an unseen weight. It begins subtly, as if you could feel a storm coming before the first black clouds appeared. It seems as if something fundamental has been stripped away in persistent grief, something that is beyond the realm of a restful night's sleep or a hopeful morning. It doesn't roar; instead, it lingers steadily into the hours until it's hard to recall what it was like to live without that tying knot.

It accumulates throughout the course of the days, a quiet burden that clings to the mind. The melancholy is accompanied by an odd sense of physical, emotional, and cerebral tiredness. Thoughts no longer move as they once did; they slow down as if walking through mud, constrained by the weight that permeates every strategy and aspiration. Laughter becomes a faint echo before being absorbed by the underlying sadness. Even happy memories seem far away, as if one were seeing someone else's life rather than their own. This melancholy becomes ingrained, blending into every minute of everyday life until even the recollection of joy is hazy.

This grief has a certain familiarity that defies explanation. It is now a method of perceiving and understanding the world rather than merely a feeling. Happy times are just momentary breaks in an otherwise constant hum of sadness, pauses in a soundtrack of grief, and do not eradicate it. When friends reach out, there's a desire to connect and experience a spark that brings back memories of who you used to be. However, even when they are together, there remains a gap, as if an imperceptible wall keeps that bond from developing fully. Everything is altered by this melancholy, which robs life of its vitality by making colors drab and sounds hollow.

SIMPLE PLEASURES THAT previously sparked an interest are often hollowed out by this grief. It obscures the comfort of a well-known fragrance, the warmth of a beloved song, and the beauty of a sunset. Conversations become cold, achievements seem meaningless, and food loses its savor. With each day carving a deeper groove, it widens the gap between who you are and the person you want to be. It casts doubt on everything, making every accomplishment seem like a coincidence and every setback an indication of some alleged weakness. Its words are pernicious, rewriting your history and influencing how you see yourself until you believe that this weight has always been a part of who you are.

There is no sensation of relief from the silent weight. It clings to every conversation, every memory, every idea. It rests on the chest, scarcely noticeable at first, but it gradually becomes larger and presses down more forcefully until breathing becomes difficult. There is a sensation of weight in the morning that only becomes worse as the hours go by. Even little things like getting dressed, preparing breakfast, and leaving the home seem like huge undertakings. The day is approaching, and every minute drags on, requiring energy that is almost unattainable. The body itself begins to react to this melancholy by retaining a weight that doesn't go away, a muscular pain, and a lethargy that sleep doesn't alleviate.

Routine so turns into survival, a list of tasks to do in order to survive the day, crossed off with no sense of accomplishment. Step by step, sometimes in a daze, and other times intensely conscious of the emptiness each action brings, you make your way through it. There is simply the comfort of a little silence and a sense of being just a little less; there is no joy in accomplishment or pride in advancement. But the melancholy lingers, infiltrating once again, like an unwanted visitor who won't go. As if the air itself has thickened and is resisting every movement, it colors even the banal, transforming the most routine duties into enormous undertakings.

THIS WEIGHT IS FOLLOWED like a shadow by isolation. There is a feeling of separation and disconnection even in the presence of other people. Their laughing seems far away, their pleasure strange. It seems like everyone else is in a separate universe where happiness comes naturally, and the environment is louder, brighter, and too fast-paced. Socializing becomes into a show, when every laugh and grin seems forced and disconnected from one's inner feelings. Thus, you retreat into a calm seclusion that seems safer but no less burdensome, protecting what little energy you have left. It takes energy to connect, and you think that energy would be better used just to get by each day.

However, there's also a certain comfort in this isolation. When there is no need to act, grin, or pretend, the world becomes smaller and easier to handle. However, there is a restlessness to it, a want for connection that grief puts just out of reach, a longing for something more than the quiet. Every social encounter seems like a tightrope walk because of the duality of requiring alone while yearning for connection. The grief that implies you're somehow different, undeserving, and a stranger in your own life is nourished by even the tiniest rejection or the slightest indication of indifference.

But below it all, there's a portion that dimly, whisperily, recalls what it was like to live without this burden. Deep down, that voice challenges the sadness's permanency and nudges you to seek out and look for solutions to overcome it. Every little action and choice to go on turns into a revolt and a reclamation of a self that this melancholy seeks to obliterate. Every effort, no matter how little, to fight the weight and look for light, even if it only lasts a short while, has strength.

THE VOICE OF DEPRESSION is unrelenting, steady, and persistent, yet it is not the only one. It's accompanied by a whisper that expresses hope for a day when happiness won't be a thing of the past and when the burden will be lifted. Offering glimmers of what life may be beyond the melancholy, that whisper battles through the shadows. Although it isn't loud or aggressive, it is there, resilient, and just waiting for an opportunity to blossom so that it may draw you out of the quiet and into a world where colors are restored and life begins to take form once again. That whisper contains the courage to face another day, to bear the burden, to resist the melancholy, and to look for a way ahead, even if it is hesitant.

The Physical Toll of Mental Pain

A tiredness that drags everything inward like a falling star is an unseen weight that gnaws at the body. This is not your typical fatigue or a passing pain that will go away with rest or sleep. Even when the body is scarcely moving, the muscles and joints feel as if they have been dragged through days of relentless labor. Simple activities become labors that consume energy meant for survival as the body slacks under the quiet weight of mental anguish.

As if carrying the weight of unseen stones, the shoulders droop. Headaches come on suddenly, like a jolt of strain that may shatter the skull itself. A continuous, gradual pressure builds up around the temples and the back of the neck, spreading downward. It pulsates with a constant reminder of anguish, sometimes drumming in sync with each pulse, and other times sitting silently, like a passenger. Because this tightness isn't only caused by strained muscles, it's also tightly coiled with every worried thought and every ounce of grief that won't go away, so no amount of stretching or massage will break the knot.

The weight seems to rest on the heart itself. Like a warning siren, anxiety infiltrates the blood, causing it to race irrationally and pound into the chest. In a language that only the body can comprehend, the beat then falters and descends into a sluggish, hollow thud that reminds you of nothingness. And it seems like the core is being progressively worn down by this cycle, which consists of bursts of terror followed by lulls of tiredness, draining vitality from every breath and pulse.

EVERY SYSTEM IS WEAKENED by mental suffering. The appetite fluctuates greatly. Food might taste like ash on some days, and the mere concept of eating can be too taxing. A vague discomfort that gnaws but doesn't demand takes the place of hunger, as if the body had also come to terms with quiet. On other days, the mind turns to tastes, textures, and the act of eating itself for solace. It's an effort to satisfy a hunger fueled by feelings much more intense than bodily need, a void that food cannot satisfy. Regardless of amount or flavor, nothing is satisfactory. As a reminder of the toll the mind has on the body, the stomach contracts, sometimes feeling empty and other times feeling heavy, as if it is digesting stones.

Once a haven, sleep becomes a battleground. Nights blend together, each one burdened by persistent thoughts. Hours pass, and each one is accompanied by a pain in the body, a tightness that intensifies as daylight draws closer. Finally, sleep arrives, but it comes in snatched moments that are insufficient to heal. Every morning is dragged through with a weariness that goes deeper than sleep alone, and eyes open with a heaviness that seems like it's ingrained in the bones. With the body taking the burden of each restless hour, rest becomes more of a battle than an escape.

The act of breathing itself becomes difficult. The chest feels constricted, as if melancholy had thickened the air itself. Every breath seems insufficient and shallow, never quite filling the lungs to their full potential. There are times when it seems as if the body has forgotten how to breathe correctly, and it briefly and shallowly gasps for air before settling back into its controlled rhythm. A subtle sense of terror persists, a hint that something is off, and a persistent undercurrent of uneasiness permeates every breath. It is as if the body recalls a moment when breathing was effortless and natural, but today it is burdened by an unsaid force.

EVEN THE SLIGHTEST motions cause energy to diminish. The pressure of daily chores has caused muscles that formerly powered through the day to hurt, as if they were carrying an unseen load that was too great to handle. It seems more difficult to walk, lift, and even stand, as if the body is objecting to the mental burden that has been entrenched. Everything is grounded in slowness as fatigue spreads across the limbs, a leaden tiredness that seeps from the toes to the fingers. Every movement seems laborious and calculated, like struggling through water, and every step requires energy that isn't there.

The skin becomes very sensitive. The slightest touch of fabric, a hand's pressure, or even the weight of clothes seems magnified, causing nerves to prickle as if to convey inside anguish. As if the body's defenses have weakened under the stress, little aches become more intense and commonplace feelings become raw. Even the temperature seems odd; heat stays longer, and cold shivers penetrate deeper. The body reacts as if it's not in sync, as though it's responding to an unrelenting distress signal.

THEN THERE ARE THE sporadic aches, such as the slow throb behind the eyes, the sudden pains in the side, or the previously absent knee soreness. Like ripples on the surface of something deeper and indefinable, they rise and fall in unpredictable ways. These aches serve solely as reminders of the body's link to the mental turmoil; they provide no explanations or hints. They become a part of life's landscape, suggesting that there is something going on under the surface. Every pain and discomfort may be traced back to a mental strain that strains every bodily fiber.

Digestion becomes erratic, responding to each emotional upswing and downs. Stomachs churn on emptiness or cramp suddenly, reflecting mental turmoil. On some days, food seems heavy and hardly breaks down, as if the body is fighting against hunger. Other times, nausea takes over, an imperceptible reaction to feelings that are too strong to communicate in any other way. The stomach, often referred to as the "second brain," seems to mirror every anxiety and shadow the mind casts.

Every day seems like a struggle against these feelings, these reminders that mental suffering is not limited to the mind. It stretches out and takes hold of the body so tightly that there is no way out. Things slow down, ideas get confused, and the pain, exhaustion, and dyspnea all come together as tangible evidence of an internal battle that goes unspoken.

CHAPTER 2
IDENTIFYING AND CHALLENGING NEGATIVE THOUGHT PATTERNS

THOUGHTS HAVE THE ABILITY to cling tightly and weave themselves into a pattern of self-criticism, uncertainty, and recurrent blame. They come subtly, often sneaking in under the pretense of facts. thoughts that seem innocuous at first, such as brief periods of reflection or anxiety. They proliferate, erecting imperceptible barriers that impede clear vision of reality. Each one encircles the mind, diverting attention from the obvious and directing it toward the gloomy or unsolved.

Automatic thoughts—those fast, reflexive responses to anything that doesn't seem quite right—often take the lead. Perhaps a casual remark is replayed and then abruptly transformed into a secret judgment or a personal shortcoming. A perceived offense creates a fissure in self-worth, and someone's quiet turns into rejection. These initially harmless emotions turn into the fundamental elements of negativity that mold the mental terrain and establish the default mood for all that comes after. Like falling dominoes in the brain's inner tempest, they set off a chain reaction, one idea after another.

It takes silent attention to identify these patterns. It involves capturing the idea in its initial instant, seeing the precise words it uses, the sharpness of its tone, and the way it steers feelings in a certain direction. Rather of ignoring it or allowing it to become the reality, you confront it and analyze the little narrative it attempts to convey. When the automatic strength behind each idea is taken away, it begins to take on a new appearance. Once accepted at face value, the criticism has now devolved into a collection of phrases attempting to establish themselves in inappropriate contexts.

THE NEXT STEP IS TO challenge these ideas—a process of doubting what seemed definite at first. You question rather than agree. "Does this idea accurately represent the circumstances?" What evidence supports or contradicts this idea outside of this thought? That little adjustment in viewpoint transforms everything, much like focusing a lens to see beyond the haze of negativity. The idea contracts, revealing itself as a transient concept that lacks substance until allowed to solidify. With every inquiry, the idea falters and is overthrown by a reality that shows through the hazy mask of pessimism.

Assumptions, such as the negative tendency to see things in shades of gray or to assume the worse, are the foundation of negative ideas. They weave together anxieties of failure, rejection, and insignificance to construct stories of worst-case situations. Prepared to see what it anticipates, the mind begins to look everywhere for evidence to support these expectations, creating narratives that support the same ideas that caused the damage. A new narrative emerges when these presumptions are identified early on and dismantled before they become ingrained. All of a sudden, the mind stops imagining what may go wrong and instead sits in the here and now, watching objectively, making space for less dramatic alternatives.

Here, self-compassion often seems far away, as if treating oneself with kindness were an alien practice. However, this is crucial—a habit that starts to change the whole conversation once it is accepted. Every negative idea is an opportunity to choose a softer understanding, a more kind reaction. Instead of criticizing yourself, try talking to a friend who is having difficulties and showing them the same tolerance and understanding. Self-compassion enables you to see your ideas as transient guests, there to educate rather than to condemn. Over time, they loosen their hold and become a part of the education rather than the condemnation.

It becomes an exercise of perseverance to break the habit of ruminating, like keeping watch at a gate where ideas attempt to enter and remain unchecked. Rumination causes the mind to replay every perceived error or imperfection in great detail, leading to never-ending cycles of rehashing. Everything comes into focus around a single, black point as each cycle becomes tighter. Ruminating just strengthens the conviction in one's perceived shortcomings and feeds an endless delusion; it doesn't fix anything. Every time you find yourself in a rut, do something tiny, like get up, move, or write something down. Anything to interrupt the pattern and divert the thoughts.

PUTTING LABELS ON IDEAS as they come to mind creates a feeling of separation. Take note of the idea and label it as a concern, a doubt, or a self-critical thought. You put it outside of yourself by labeling it, making it a distinct thing that doesn't determine your reality. To perceive it for what it is—one little bit of mental noise among millions that come and go—this act of naming creates enough distance. With each label added, each idea becomes lighter and less significant, no longer disguised as a secret reality but rather as a fleeting urge that can be released.

The background of these ideas is shaped by beliefs, which often provide the groundwork for all of the mental speech. Old beliefs that are accepted without examination begin to influence patterns and provide frameworks for concepts of potential, value, and competence. They provide a standard by which all other things are evaluated and are often acquired from prior experiences. The level of inquiry increases here. Examine the belief that underlies the idea rather than just the thinking itself. "What makes me think this? What evidence backs up or refutes this belief? With every response, a new component of the negative framework falls away, making room for ideas that are not predicated on self-criticism.

Gratitude practice may seem pointless, like an effort to hide rust, but when done intentionally, it helps the mind find equilibrium. Being grateful causes one's attention to change from what is missing to what is still there and functioning. Recognizing one item that seems significant every day is a simple gesture. It seems forced at first, like trying to find a glimmer of truth in a desolate place. However, each acknowledgment gives the opposing viewpoint more weight, bringing the equation into balance and teaching the mind to consider all sides of any given circumstance rather than focusing just on the bad.

BY EXTERNALIZING UNPLEASANT ideas, you may use another tool to analyze each one as if it were someone else's. Put it in writing, read it out loud, and even debate it from an outsider's point of view. This action takes away the personal stake, allowing you to see the idea as if it were a play scenario rather than a judgment on your personality. With this perspective, the idea is no longer an unquestionable reality but rather a hypothesis, a theory to be tested. Its grip loosens with every analysis, exposing the prejudice it concealed.

The hold of negative beliefs gradually becomes lessened by disputing, naming, reframing, and asking questions. The mind starts to rewrite its own story after being constrained by recurring scripts of skepticism and criticism. Thought by thought, it creates a new script, one that is open to possibilities beyond what fear and grief originally commanded and is not rooted in uncompromising self-criticism. The goal is to deprive negative ideas of their previous strength, not to deny their existence. Clarity, a calmer mental space where ideas are no longer free to rule, and a feeling of agency that had before been gone are what are left.

The Cycle of Negative Self-Talk

Like slow-moving water eroding stone, self-talk permeates everything and shapes the mental landscape. It infiltrates every thought, establishing a rhythm and a constant murmur that never stops playing in the background. The cycle starts innocently with a little inward remark, maybe a minor criticism or a mutter of dissatisfaction. Then it becomes stronger. It feeds on frustrations, fears, and memories of previous failures, entangling people in a web of doubt and self-blame. Every murmur becomes louder, harsher, and more damning. Before long, this silent discussion shapes vision, corrupts experience, and leaves little space for anything other than harsh criticism and fault-finding.

With every turn, a negative idea spirals into another, turning little setbacks into evidence of failure and disappointment into proof of incompetence. An internal storm of criticism and irritation may rage for days, weeks, or even years due to this subtle kind of mental gravity that draws everything inward. What began as a fleeting idea or a little self-doubt grows into something comprehensive. Like a prison made of words that only the mind can hear, it produces patterns that seem unbreakable.

Every little error or perceived slight turns into a building brick, giving the inner voice another opportunity to repeat, "See? There's more evidence. Errors become shortcomings; ambiguity becomes vulnerability. As the prosecutor, witness, and judge in a skewed trial, the mind turns into its own jury, gathering and assembling evidence. Thoughts become into rigid, unyielding laws that require constant evidence of accomplishment, value, or validation yet never provide it. With each movement, word, and deed, the harsh sentence serves as a continual reminder of one's shortcomings.

PERFECTIONISM IS AT its core, a root that feeds the system as a whole. Perfectionism sets unrealistic standards that no one can achieve and views even the smallest flaw as a failure. One little error turns into a character defect, a manifestation of an innate shortcoming. Using perfectionism as a benchmark, the mind continuously reassesses itself, scrutinizing each action and thought to pinpoint areas where it has failed. Nothing ever achieves "good enough" in this cycle as the goal is always shifting, becoming more taunting, unachievable, and out of reach.

The loop grows increasingly self-fulfilling the more it repeats. The inner voice demands impossible, observes the inevitable failure that ensues, and then exploits it as evidence of its own insufficiency. The mind finds a way to minimize their importance and disregard them, as if nothing ever fully measures up, so even outward achievements are unable to stop the pattern. Failures are emphasized and successes are written off as flukes, reinforcing the idea that nothing is ever really right.

Catching these beliefs early on, before they have a chance to spread, is the first step in breaking the cycle. It involves seeing the remark as it emerges, experiencing the pull of self-doubt, and realizing that it is not an actual fact but rather a part of a well-worn, recognizable screenplay. Early detection allows you to face it, challenge its veracity, and deprive it of the burden it attempts to bear. Breaking the loop entails questioning the strength of the concept and determining if it has any truth other than the self-imposed condemnation it conveys.

SELF-COMPASSION, A soft voice that interrupts the cycle, even for a little while, causes a tiny change. This voice only gives patience and empathy instead of rushing in with lofty pronouncements. It turns inward and says, "You're allowed to be imperfect." The cycle becomes weaker with every act of kindness. The script begins to shift, the prosecuting ideas seem more reasonable, and the inner judge loses ground. Where self-blame had previously reigned, self-compassion fills the voids with kindness where criticism had previously been the norm.

Breaking the cycle also involves turning attention outside and away from the self-analysis that feeds negative discourse. By interacting with the outside world via an activity, a discussion, or a simple chore, the mind's energy is diverted and directed toward something constructive. The act stops the ideas from repeating themselves incessantly and places value elsewhere, but it does not reject or conceal them. Thoughts lose speed and dissipate without fuel whenever the mind changes attention. This act, which turns self-focus into a soft external presence, becomes simpler with experience.

Small deeds of self-compassion further break the loop. It involves little adjustments to the way ideas are permitted to reside in the mind rather than a complete makeover. As the mind starts searching for things to be thankful for, practicing thankfulness provides a counterbalance to self-criticism. These actions rewire the reaction, substituting peaceful times with severe judgments. Small flashes of brightness and reminders that things don't have to be flawless or fit some impossibly rigid mold in order to be valuable are brought about by gratitude.

Slowly, self-talk changes to something kinder and more kind. What used to condemn now watches. There is now a chance for self-acceptance when there was previously just criticism. A new pattern emerges with every little instance of defiance against the critical voice. A nicer conversation with oneself, which at first seemed unattainable, becomes a reality, a place where the mind learns to sit without turning every idea into an assault.

RESILIENCE INCREASES when this change occurs. Instead of tightening like a trap, the self-talk loop now relaxes, making space for development, errors, and silent triumphs. After being taught to critique, the mind starts to perceive things more broadly, embracing flaws and appreciating achievements without feeling the need to minimize or discount them. Self-talk starts to change into a voice of support, an ally instead of an enemy, one that acknowledges difficulties without passing judgment or using blunders as a weapon.

There is now room for every thinking to evolve, moving from judgment to neutrality or even acceptance. The mind becomes lighter, letting go of the urge for continual criticism and discovering serenity even in flaws. The once-unrelenting cycle begins to break down, making room for something gentler to take root and allowing ideas to come and go without being attached to the heart.

Rewriting Inner Narratives

Ideas take on a life of their own, becoming heavier and more definite until they seem indestructible and merge into what seems to be the sole reality. Reality is framed with a definite, uncompromising gravity by the tales the mind creates, which turn into the walls and shadows. Every phrase is well-known, every plot twist is anticipated, and the story moves along so naturally. It seems more and more plausible every day, as if any other viewpoint would be untrue. Your inner voice takes on the roles of storyteller, critic, and judge. Its script is harsh and full of skepticism, and it speaks in a monotone that excludes all other voices. Every phrase is repeated, narrating a story of scarcity, squandered opportunities, and failure. You bear it with you, a load of words, something you know but don't want.

However, what if the script can be altered? Rewriting entails paying more attention, carefully reading the lines, and identifying any incorrect presumptions that may be concealed between them. Catchphrases like "always" and "never," which sound so solid but seldom stand up to inspection, are what it's all about. It's important to pause before believing the mind's stale conclusions since they are just one viewpoint and not the only one. When you begin to doubt each sentence, probe its veracity, and contest its authority, the rewriting process starts.

REPETITION GIVES STORIES strength, while interruption weakens them. Think of a single thought: "I'm not good enough." It defines the failure narrative and serves as the story's anchor. But if you flip it over and look at it from a different perspective, the defect is visible. What is "not good enough" in comparison to? To whom? By what criteria? Every query rips away the narrative's edges, allowing light to seep in. It reveals the idea as a flimsy structure supported by presumptions that break down when examined closely. In order to break the narrative, its blind strength must be removed and replaced with a question mark, a soft pause that asks, "Is this truly true?"

Every tale has a framework, and the majority of internal narratives are based on recurring patterns. They use the same strategies, making snap decisions, holding to recollections of previous errors, and latching to times of uncertainty. The ground changes as these patterns are recognized. It's similar like reading the same book over and then realizing you already know the story. Every time the same scene—self-doubt, self-blame, regret—occurs, you recognize it for what it is: a reenactment of an old chapter rather than a new discovery. With every acknowledgment, the pattern loses its hold, the cycle becomes less rigid, and room is created for something new.

This revamp is a slow, piecemeal process rather than an abrupt makeover. By experimenting with fresh words and phrases, it seems as if the mind is finally beginning to release its hold on long-held ideas. The story may become adaptable rather than inflexible and subject to changes. Every time a severe verdict is rendered, a new script is made feasible. The statement changes from "I failed" to "I learned" or "I tried." Words like "sometimes" and "never" replace "always" and "never," smoothing the edges. It ultimately comes down to developing kinder language that accepts errors without denouncing them.

COMPASSION TAKES THE lead in rewriting, taking the place of criticism. Self-compassion creates fresh words and phrases that allow for development rather than stifling it. It provides words like "There's room to try again" or "This doesn't define me." Compassion allows the narrative to grow and develop without a harsh ending. It is a recognition of humanity's imperfection and prevents the intellect from imposing judgment each time anything goes wrong. The story moves from final to open-ended, from stiff to flexible, with every good word.

Finding the inner narrator's voice is about learning to offer a counterpoint, to create balance, rather than eradicating any negative feelings or self-doubt. It's being rewritten to prevent pessimistic ideas from taking precedence and to make the narrative less depressing and hopeless. It involves inserting new lines that provide perspective and opportunity into the script. A rewrite doesn't eliminate all negative ideas; instead, it provides new voices, gentler ones that provide balance, soften the tone, and bring reason where there was just judgment. Perhaps the inner narrator declares, "You'll never succeed," but a new voice responds, "One failure doesn't decide my future."

Choice is at the heart of this revision. There is an opportunity to choose each line, to determine what remains and what is removed, rather than reverting to the previous storyline. There is a chance to expose ideas to the light, to review them like an editor would, and to remove any sections that are just harmful. The old story eventually loses its impact and is replaced with one that is truthful and sympathetic, one that accepts reality without placing undue emphasis on it.

SELF-TRUST, A SHAKY but steady confidence, builds as the new tale takes shape. Every time a line is rewritten, the mind gains confidence in its capacity to perceive clearly, to see negativity when it arises, and to gently steer itself back on course. This self-confidence serves as a solid base, a silent assurance that endures failures without crumbling. Knowing that no chapter is ever complete and that the tale may be rewritten if necessary enables the mind to go patiently.

Reality is shaped by language, and the mind may affect how it perceives the world and itself by carefully selecting words. It becomes feasible to interpret obstacles as milestones, to perceive failures as teaching opportunities, and to view flaws with compassion. Every well selected phrase creates a fresh perspective and a new way of living that doesn't burden but uplifts, doesn't constrain but liberates.

CHAPTER 3
NURTURING EMOTIONAL RESILIENCE AND SELF-COMPASSION

WHILE LIFE IS FRAYING at the edges, resilience quietly keeps the mind together. It is often overlooked. It's the part of you that rises even when exhaustion sets in, the instinct that urges, "Get up." But resilience doesn't yell; it doesn't cry triumph in the face of defeat. Rather, it infuses periods of vulnerability with power, encouraging you to take a breath and to press on even when it would seem simpler to give up. Additionally, emotional resilience provides a softer landing for the mind's freefall as life's burdens bear down on it. Through failures, the midst of difficulties, and the gentle self-talk that follows a misstep, this resilience develops over time. It is developed rather than inherited, and it becomes stronger every time you choose to continue going in the face of adversity.

Building resilience is enduring suffering without losing your composure and enduring feelings that seem too intense to manage, knowing that they will pass. Every difficult day adds a layer, and every setback adds a thread. Being resilient means being able to experience sorrow and suffering fully and allow them to pass without redefining who you are. It does not imply being immune to them. Think of it as a muscle that has been built through strain and becomes stronger with every demand. Every time patience is put to the test and bravery seems to be waning, resilience increases and turns weakness into silent strength.

AWAITING IN THE BACKDROP is self-compassion. Kindness is what keeps resilience together, and it's the voice that intervenes when self-criticism becomes loudest. Self-compassion gently but firmly asks you to embrace your humanity and make peace with imperfection by looking at the rough edges and the times you want to hide and saying, "This too belongs." Self-compassion reaches out and provides consolation without being overbearing if resilience is lacking. When combined, they provide a strong foundation that neither minimizes nor allows suffering to impede progress.

Self-compassion and resilience are two factors that reinforce one another. While self-compassion makes the ride more tolerable, resilience keeps you standing. They are there when you make mistakes, when guilt starts to seep in, and when the critic tries to take control. You may accept errors without feeling guilty when you have compassion. This small act of compassion changes the old habit of self-punishment and replaces it with tolerance, saying, "This is part of learning." Resilience develops during that wait, providing you with the willpower to persevere—not by coercion, but by comprehension.

Being self-compassionate is treating oneself with the same consideration as you would a friend. Imagine using gentler language when you talk to yourself and forgiving yourself for your errors just as easily as you would someone else. Compassion intervenes when you make a mistake, reminding you that everyone makes mistakes and that development is never linear. Self-compassion views errors as a necessary part of the process rather than as something to be indulged. It makes you answerable without passing judgment, allowing you to try again without feeling guilty. Resilience emerges when self-compassion takes hold, bolstered by the freedom to develop without worrying about unrelenting judgment.

RESILIENCE OFTEN SEEMS like a decision, a conscious act of persevering in the face of adversity. It serves as a reminder that there is no set course in life and that failures do not spell doom. By providing perspective, resilience enables you to see difficulties as parts of a larger narrative. Resilient people don't make snap judgments when things go awry. Rather, it serves as a reminder to stop, collect your power, and remember that you are not yet at your best. Resilience provides the strength, and self-compassion provides the insight. Together, they create a path ahead that, one cautious step at a time, rebuilds you rather than shatters you.

These traits are developed in the little things, in the silent times when resilience pushes you ahead and self-compassion sustains you. Imagine waking up every day without the desire to control every consequence, allowing yourself to live instead of fighting. Being resilient implies being flexible and able to adjust to life's curveballs without losing your essence. You make an unwritten commitment to yourself to try again and to go on gracefully even in the absence of assurance. And when resilience takes root, it creates a life that overcomes adversity rather than escaping it.

Developing these traits turns into a daily routine that involves accepting failures and overcoming obstacles without harboring resentment against oneself. You may start by acknowledging the little triumphs—each day encountered, every challenge met with hope. Resilience develops over time via overcoming obstacles and being nice to oneself throughout the most trying times, not through victories. Self-compassion turns into the voice that strikes a balance between resilience and softens the blows, allowing you to breathe and try again without being held back by your previous mistakes.

BEING RESILIENT CHANGES how you see yourself—from someone who has been beaten by life to someone who is capable of facing it head-on. Additionally, self-compassion alters the way you speak to yourself, allowing kindness to take the place of criticism and seeing imperfections as a necessary component of the process rather than a sign of inferiority. Together, they build a foundation that keeps you afloat, one that experiences suffering without allowing it to break you, one that recognizes errors without allowing them to define you. Resilience becomes the power that keeps self-compassion in place, and self-compassion becomes the warmth that keeps resilience going.

Resilience and self-compassion are ultimately partners on the trip that help you get there, not final destinations. They create a route that views adversity as a teaching opportunity, embraces failure as a necessary component of learning, and allows you to grow without losing your tender sides. They support one another with every step, building a life that can endure adversity without being closed off, one that harbors suffering without allowing it to become resentful. This route enables you to go with resilience softened by compassion and strength tempered by kindness, establishing a way of being that doesn't minimize hardship but rather thrives on it.

Building Emotional Resilience in Everyday Life

Developing resilience is similar to piecing together little, everyday actions of bravery to become something robust enough to withstand life's unforeseen setbacks. Imagine every action, every silent choice to confront discomfort instead of avoiding it, as a thread sewn into a fabric of strength. It isn't about arming oneself against the outside world or preparing for impact. It's about developing a softness that endures through difficult times and a flexibility that takes stress without breaking.

Resilience in daily life starts with the seemingly little occurrences. It involves choosing to pause before responding and to take a deep breath when irritation flares. Resilience begins to develop when one recognizes an inclination and resists it. These brief pauses allow for the processing of emotions and allow them to flow through without getting carried away. It is at these times of self-control that resilience develops ingrained in your internal structure, influencing how you respond to stress and setbacks.

Every day is an opportunity to develop resilience, to experience emotions without letting them control you. Small acts of self-awareness, such as checking in with your emotions and understanding what's causing them, help create a mental space where resilience may flourish. Facing the unpleasant turns into an endurance workout, a means of reminding yourself, "This is difficult, but I can handle it." It is a haven that accommodates both suffering and progress, where emotions are let to exist without controlling conduct.

When difficulties arise, resilience is derived from these regular mindfulness exercises and the power that comes from handling little annoyances without losing your composure. It doesn't imply that the difficulties don't cause you pain or anxiety. It indicates that you have established a solid foundation that will last, a network of little decisions that will enable you to continue in the face of adversity. Additionally, resilience becomes stronger, more ingrained in your identity, and thicker every time you persevere through a challenging situation.

IMAGINE CHOOSING TO ground yourself every morning and start the day with a steady activity, such as a practice, a thought, or a breath. These routines, the habits you develop to begin each day with intention, foster resilience. It might be a quick meditation, a little period of stillness, or even just stretching. Every morning routine serves as a reminder to your mind that, despite all that the day may throw at you, there is a core that remains constant. These instances provide a silent reassurance and serve as a reminder that resilience is always there and prepared to help you through challenging times.

A life devoid of adversity does not cultivate resilience. It emerges from overcoming adversity and deciding to keep going, little by little. In daily life, it may be found in the simple act of getting back up after each setback and in accepting misfortunes without harboring grudges. Resilience is not about erecting barriers against suffering, but about being ready to sit with it, confront it, and acknowledge its existence without allowing it to control your decisions. It's an internal attitude that says, "I can be with this without losing myself." Resilience finds strength in every little setback, changing and growing with each encounter.

To be emotionally resilient, you must be nice to yourself and treat your inner life with the same consideration that you would show someone else. This entails recognizing when you are being harsh and judgmental of yourself, when you feel lost or insufficient, and talking to yourself patiently instead. Resilience is seeing each setback as a teaching opportunity and a method of improving one's understanding of oneself rather than punishing oneself for it. Resilience develops at these times when you let go of the need to be flawless and accept yourself as you are, replacing self-blame with self-acceptance.

EVERY DAY OFFERS A fresh chance to strengthen resilience by practicing self-compassion during stressful situations. Life will put your patience and commitment to the test, but resilience doesn't need perfect endurance. It requires perseverance and the resolve to wake up each day and try again. Resilient people approach setbacks with a calm curiosity and see them as a necessary component of a bigger journey. Resilience turns setbacks into fuel by realizing that they are a necessary component of progress, and each obstacle becomes a step toward becoming a more resilient, stronger version of oneself.

Resilience serves as a reminder that endurance, not resistance, is what makes you strong when you're feeling uncertain. It's the capacity to continue breathing, walking, and attempting even when the way forward is uncertain. Being resilient is a process of developing your ability to confront life with an open mind and without ignoring its challenges; it is not something you can acquire. It turns into a method of getting around that allows you to fully experience and feel things without losing yourself in the midst of them.

THINK OF RESILIENCE as a constant pulse that keeps you rooted when things go wrong, a calm resolve. It's an inside warmth, a light that becomes brighter every time you decide to stay going and confront the difficult things instead of running away from them. This resilience only has to be steady; it doesn't need to be loud or aggressive. In daily life, resilience is developed via little decisions like trying again, forgiving oneself, and embracing each day with the ability to handle any situation that arises.

Leaning into life with an openness to learning, adapting, and accepting whatever comes up—no matter how uncertain—is the foundation of building resilience. It is the act of putting yourself first, even in the tiniest ways, and building a foundation that is resilient enough to withstand adversity and pliable enough to bend without breaking. Resilience is developed throughout daily struggles, becoming stronger each time you face a challenging situation head-on. It involves approaching every moment with openness, allowing resilience to develop by acceptance rather than opposition, and being prepared to remain in the present no matter what happens.

Practicing Self-Compassion and Kindness

A route of tenderness that breaks through the cacophony of harsh judgment and self-criticism is revealed by engaging in self-compassion and kindness practices. It involves creating an atmosphere inside oneself where kindness flourishes and the natural tendency to criticize oneself changes into a supportive voice. Imagine getting up every day with a heart prepared to accept your flaws and treat yourself with the same compassion as you would a close friend going through a difficult time. In the chilly recesses of the mind, where uncertainty and hopelessness often reside, this exercise brings warmth.

Begin by just acknowledging your emotions. Recognize your feelings of melancholy or dissatisfaction without passing judgment. Every emotion has a history and a purpose. Invite these feelings to remain for a little rather than rushing to ignore or conceal them. Imagine having an open ear and a place to discuss your burdens while sitting across from an old friend. Being present facilitates the flow of knowledge and builds a bridge to compassion.

Small, kind decisions made in the present are how self-compassion shows itself in day-to-day living. When confronted with errors, a gentle murmur of acceptance may make all the difference instead of harsh remarks. Resilience is strengthened by the slogan, "I'm human; I'm learning." Every setback is an opportunity to learn and develop. Accept the discomfort that comes with making errors and let them serve as stepping stones instead of roadblocks. A fresh layer of kindness envelops your soul each time self-compassion takes the place of judgment.

THE ORDINARY MAY BECOME spectacular via the establishment of compassion rituals. Think about the impact that a few minutes spent just on self-care may have. These activities, whether it's making a hot cup of tea, going for a leisurely stroll in the outdoors, or engaging in a beloved pastime, are soul-nourishing. They serve as a reminder that self-care starts at home. By making time for these activities, the mind is trained to connect self-love with commonplace events, resulting in a rhythm of compassion that is calming and organic.

Consider the story that is always playing in your head, the incessant internal conversation. Change the tone of this discussion to one of compassion by substituting positive statements with negative ones. Anchors amid the storm include "I am enough," "I am worthy of love," and "I am doing my best." Let these words remain steadfast when the winds of doubt roar. By repeating them throughout difficult circumstances, you may reshape your self-perception and sense of value by integrating compassion into your own thinking.

INTERACTING WITH OTHER people may improve your compassion practice. Sharing vulnerabilities with close friends fosters a network of support and unrestricted empathy. It's simpler to show compassion for oneself when you realize that other people have comparable difficulties. Connection-building conversations give you perspective and serve as a reminder that nobody travels this path alone. By sharing your stories, you perpetuate a culture of compassion in which being vulnerable turns into a strength and a lovely thread that unites others.

Remind yourself of your compassion whenever you start to feel lonely. Think back to instances when you were compassionate toward others, even if it was only by listening to them or providing assistance. Remember how wonderful it was to encourage someone else? You get the same energy in return, serving as a reminder that generosity is cyclical. It spreads, entwining your heart with those around you and enhancing the good effects of every little deed.

It's critical to make room for self-forgiveness while developing self-compassion. Errors and blunders are temporary events in the vast scheme of things; they are not permanent fixtures. After you've admitted your mistakes, let go of the guilt with grace. Healing is facilitated by forgiveness, which makes space for development and comprehension. Imagine forgiveness as a soft wind that blows through the mind, removing trash and making room for new ideas.

ACKNOWLEDGING THE VALUE of mindfulness is another aspect of starting this self-compassion path. Being mindful encourages you to be in the moment and to feel your feelings without passing judgment. Accept emotions as a natural aspect of the human experience, whether they be grief, worry, or rage. Noticing their existence without holding on to or pushing them away, observe them as clouds move across the sky. By cultivating a feeling of calm, this practice helps you respond to difficulties with compassion instead of fear or annoyance.

Eliminating challenging emotions is not the aim of the self-compassion journey. It's about learning to live with them instead. Accept the intricacy of your emotional terrain and realize that pleasure, sorrow, and all points in between combine to form a diverse tapestry of human experience. Give yourself permission to feel fully, understanding that every emotion has knowledge and insight that profoundly shapes who you are.

REMEMBER THAT COMPASSION may serve as a buffer when negativity starts to creep in. Seek for resources that encourage self-kindness, such as journaling, artistic expression, or exercise, rather than sinking into hopelessness. By doing these things, energy is transformed and directed toward positive and constructive endeavors. In times of darkness, each deed turns into a lighthouse that leads you back to a place of acceptance and self-love.

Developing a self-compassionate lifestyle encourages spiritual growth. It builds resilience, promoting development through hardship and cultivating a sense of adventure. A vast universe becomes available to you as you learn to be nice to yourself; every setback becomes a teaching opportunity, every difficult time a stepping stone. This gentle method changes the mental terrain, establishing a sanctuary where self-love and compassion thrive.

In the end, developing self-compassion is a lifetime process that takes time to complete. You create the foundation for a more positive connection with yourself with every deliberate act of kindness. Accept the little triumphs, the times when compassion triumphs over self-criticism, and see how they add up to something significant. You may use this practice as a basis to create a compassionate and understanding existence that will always nourish your inner heart.

CHAPTER 4
HEALING THROUGH LIFESTYLE CHANGES AND DAILY ROUTINES

ADOPTING NEW LIFESTYLE choices may lead to healing and turn everyday activities into effective partners on the path to wellbeing. Imagine that each little change in behavior serves as a step toward escaping the darkness of long-term despair. It's about creating a new way of life, one little adjustment at a time, rather than striving for perfection or a complete makeover.

Start by thinking about nutrition. Food serves as mental and physical fuel, impacting mood, energy levels, and general health. A healthy foundation is created by packing the plate full of lean meats, complete grains, and vibrant fruits and vegetables. Consider meals as chances for healing rather than just as a source of nourishment. Cooking experiments may be a fun way to interact with food and turn the kitchen into a creative and nurturing environment. Cooking turns becomes a ritual, a time to engage with the food and recognize the sustenance they provide.

Emotional stability and mental clarity are also significantly impacted by hydration. Every cell in the body runs on water, which also aids in eliminating pollutants and preserving optimum health. Reaching for a drink of water may be a quick and easy way to center yourself when you're feeling overwhelmed. It serves as a reminder that self-care starts with the fundamentals. Water may be made more exciting by adding fresh fruits or herbs, which makes staying hydrated a fun routine rather than a job.

ANOTHER CRUCIAL COMPONENT of the problem is movement. Movement raises the soul and gets the blood flowing, whether it's via a calm yoga practice, a quick stroll, or a dance session in the living room. Enjoy your body's rhythm and allow it to be a manifestation of your freedom. It has nothing to do with rigorous exercise regimens or gym subscriptions. Instead, it's about finding what makes you happy—how movement speaks to your spirit. The cycle of inactivity that often accompanies sadness may be broken by even brief spurts of exercise throughout the day.

Breathing exercises are a means of achieving immediate serenity. Concentrating on the breath may provide a haven of calm when emotions are rushing and thoughts are racing. Easy techniques that promote calm and clarity include the 4-7-8 method and deep belly breathing. Imagine releasing what no longer serves you by visualizing the inhalation of positive energy and the exhalation of negative energy. By practicing mindfulness, you become more aware and rooted in the here and now.

Developing a regular sleep schedule becomes essential. Sleep promotes healing and regeneration by revitalizing the body and mind. Make a relaxing nighttime routine a priority and create a sleeping environment that promotes relaxation. Turn down the lights, turn off the phone, and maybe listen to some relaxing music or read a nice book. The body's natural ability to wind down promotes a state of calm that prepares the body for healing sleep.

THINK ABOUT HOW SOCIAL media and technology affect day-to-day living. These platforms might help people connect, but they can also make them feel more alone and inadequate. Maintaining a healthy connection with technology may be achieved by taking breaks from displays, particularly before bed. Investigate creative and joyful pursuits like writing, sketching, or just taking in the scenery rather than sifting through feeds. You may get a much-needed break from digital distractions by reestablishing a connection with the real world.

Establishing a self-care-focused habit makes a haven in the middle of turmoil. Set aside time for pursuits that uplift your soul, such as taking a hot bath, engaging in a hobby, or spending time outside. This deliberate emphasis on taking care of yourself acts as a reminder that you deserve love and care. Set aside time every day, no matter how little, to respect your needs and wants.

Another essential component of wellbeing is social ties. Having helpful people around you may be quite relieving. Talk to one other, exchange stories, and support one another when things become difficult. Reaching out to friends or family when you're feeling lonely serves as a lifeline, letting you know you're not alone. Think about becoming involved in organizations, groups, or community events that suit your interests. This may help people feel like they belong and provide doors to real friendships.

By encouraging a feeling of awareness and presence, mindfulness exercises blend in seamlessly with everyday activities. Whether having a meal, sipping tea, or going on a stroll, living in the present moment may foster pleasure and thankfulness. Accept the little joys that are often overlooked; this exercise helps refocus attention from pessimistic ideas to gratitude for life's small joys.

INTEGRATING CREATIVITY into everyday life provides a therapeutic and expressive outlet. Creative pursuits, whether they include painting, writing, making, or playing an instrument, provide the soul a chance to express itself. Creating without criticism and allowing one's imagination to run wild has a very healing effect. Make time to investigate this aspect of yourself and let it grow in whichever way seems most appropriate.

Momentum is increased by acknowledging and applauding little accomplishments along the way. Every action, no matter how little, should be recognized. Whether it's picking a healthy meal, taking a shower, or getting out of bed, these little activities add up to a feeling of achievement. To provide a concrete reminder of progress accomplished during trying times, keep a notebook to record these victories.

Spending time in nature may be calming and restorative. The splendor of nature offers a setting for introspection and renewal. Spend some time walking outside, taking in the scenery, and feeling the earth under your feet. You feel more connected to the world around you when you take in the sounds of life, the hues of the sky, and the changing seasons. In the midst of turmoil, nature provides perspective and a sense of stability by inviting calm.

LAST BUT NOT LEAST, developing an attitude of thankfulness promotes optimism. Think about the things you value every day, whether it's a warm cup of coffee, a kind act from a complete stranger, or the sunlight streaming through your window. By directing attention away from what is missing and onto life's benefits, gratitude serves as a potent antidote to negativity.

Starting this process of altering everyday habits and lifestyle choices promotes a significant shift. It weaves self-love, self-care, and purpose into a tapestry. A new way of being that respects the complexity of the human experience while promoting hope and healing is created by every decision, every instance, and every act of compassion. A route toward a better, more satisfying life emerges through dedication to these disciplines.

The Role of Sleep and Nutrition

Nutrition and sleep are fundamental components in the pursuit of wellbeing. They establish a mutually beneficial connection that feeds the body and the mind, interacting in ways that affect mood, vitality, and mental health in general. Imagine the cycle: when one fails, the other often does too. It is a dance that influences emotional fortitude and day-to-day living.

First, let's talk about sleep. It is impossible to overestimate the value of getting enough good sleep. The body goes through a healing process every night, mending cells and digesting the events of the day. Sleep enables the brain to arrange ideas, creating space for concentration and clarity. Imagine waking up after a good night's sleep with your body and mind refreshed and prepared to take on the day. On the other hand, a sleepless night often results in lethargy, anger, and mental fog, which may spiral into a negative cycle.

Establishing a nightly routine becomes crucial to encouraging improved sleep hygiene. To let the body know it's time to relax, think about turning down the lights one hour before bed. The mind may enter a tranquil state with the aid of relaxing activities like reading a book, doing moderate yoga, or listening to relaxing music. The body starts to equate the bedroom with calm and relaxation when it becomes a haven free from pressures and interruptions.

IN TERMS OF MENTAL health, nutrition is also crucial. Our mental and physical states are both nourished by the food we eat. The brain and body are efficiently fueled by a diet high in whole foods, such as fruits, vegetables, whole grains, and lean meats. Every meal turns into a chance to feed the mind, affecting emotional stability and energy levels. Think about the relationship between food choices and emotions: a plate full of vibrant nutrients energizes, while a heavy, processed meal may cause sluggishness.

Mealtimes become rituals of gratitude as mindful eating becomes a powerful discipline. A closer relationship with food is possible when one is totally involved in the eating process. Awareness is increased by enjoying every meal and taking in the tastes, textures, and scents. This exercise improves contentment, facilitates digestion, and cultivates thankfulness.

What about the notorious link between mood swings and sugar? Although sugary foods may provide a short-term lift, they often result in a crash that leaves you exhausted and agitated. However, adding complex carbs, such as quinoa, brown rice, and oats, helps to balance blood sugar levels and gives you a consistent energy source all day. This consistency lessens the possibility of the emotional rollercoasters that might result from changes in energy levels and encourages a healthy attitude.

HYDRATION IS SHOWN as an often-overlooked hero in this investigation of nutrition and sleep. Water is essential for preserving emotional equilibrium and cerebral clarity. Fatigue, agitation, and trouble focusing may result from dehydration. Maintaining a water bottle close at hand and drinking from it throughout the day promotes the habit of keeping hydrated. Not only can adding fruits or herbs to water make it more pleasurable, but it also acts as a reminder to put self-care first.

There is growing interest in the relationship between gut health and mental wellness. A complex bacterial environment in the gut affects emotions, cognitive processes, and general health. Foods high in probiotics, such kefir, yogurt, and fermented vegetables, may help maintain a balanced gut flora. Adopting these meals may help you feel better emotionally, which might have an impact on your general health.

Understanding the effects of coffee on mood and sleep is another crucial component. Although it may seem necessary to have a cup of coffee in the morning, too much caffeine may interfere with sleep cycles and exacerbate anxiety. The secret is striking the correct balance. Choose a milder brew or herbal tea in place of one cup of coffee so that your body may flourish without the jitters.

THE BODY'S INTERNAL clock is nurtured by regular sleep and feeding schedules, which supports mood and energy stability. It's simpler to fall asleep and wake up feeling rejuvenated when you go to bed and wake up at the same time every day. In a similar vein, setting regular mealtimes keeps the body balanced by avoiding sharp swings in appetite and energy.

Stress may disrupt sleep and nutrition when it manifests. Reaching for comfort foods—those short-term solutions that provide temporary respite but leave one feeling unfulfilled later—is often the result of stress eating. It becomes crucial to raise awareness of stressors and identify substitute coping strategies. Instead of reaching for unhealthy treats, think about engaging in creative endeavors, mindfulness exercises, or physical activities. This change promotes better eating habits in addition to fostering mental well-being.

Additionally, mindfulness may significantly improve the quality of your sleep. The body and mind are prepared for sleep by techniques including gradual muscular relaxation, deep breathing, and meditation. Breaking the cycle of tension and worry that often afflict evenings, healthy sleep is made possible when the mind calms.

It requires consideration to create a sleeping-friendly atmosphere. Think about the things that promote relaxation: a cold environment, cozy bedding, and little noise. Making a to-do list or writing down problems before bed may assist those who have trouble sleeping by clearing their minds and promoting a more restful sleep.

THE FOUNDATIONS OF diet and sleep may also be strengthened by adopting a balanced lifestyle. Maintaining social relationships, getting regular exercise, and spending time outside all improve general well-being. The harmonic interaction of these components fosters a feeling of balance that permeates both eating and sleep.

It takes time and deliberate effort to raise awareness of the connection between diet and sleep. It involves trying out different approaches, identifying what works, and making necessary adjustments. Even though some days can seem more difficult than others, little, steady adjustments lead to improvement.

Sleep and diet are essential threads that weave together the fabric of mental wellness in this complex tapestry of life. Every decision—whether to emphasize restorative sleep, feed the body healthy meals, or practice mindfulness—becomes a conscious step toward recovery. Even if the route may not be straight, every effort to improve sleep and diet builds resilience and creates a safe haven where the voices of chronic depression eventually subside.

Movement, Exercise, and Mental Health

Exercise and movement serve as stimulants in the pursuit of mental health, changing the mind as well as the body. Every walk, stretch, or lift improves mood and lessens the burden of persistent depression by causing ripples in the fabric of mental health. Regaining control over one's emotions via physical exercise turns into a self-care practice.

Consider the basic activity of walking. The pulse and the rhythm of feet striking the ground combine to produce a meditative state that slows rushing thoughts. Every exhale relieves stress, and every inhalation brings in fresh air. It becomes a grounding technique as much as a means of mobility, letting the mind roam and often resulting in fresh ideas or insight.

The realm of exercise offers a multitude of options for those who want to increase their level of intensity. Everyone can find their way, whether it's via the flowing movements of yoga or the explosive energy of dancing. Whether it's the serene concentration of tai chi or the exhilarating rush of kickboxing, the joy is in figuring out what works for you. A spark that raises the soul is ignited by each modality's own approach to connecting with the body.

THE FORCE OF MOVEMENT is shown by its science. Endorphins, the feel-good chemicals that provide a natural high, are released when you exercise. It's like drawing from an inner reservoir of joy that is waiting to spill forth with every step. This biological response revives the intellect and lifts spirits, acting as a counterbalance to the fog of despair.

However, the path to mobility goes beyond the yoga studio or the gym. It brings possibilities for movement into everyday living. Stretching at work breaks, dancing in the living room, or choosing the stairs over the elevator all contribute to the tapestry of motion that permeates daily life. A feeling of success and vigor are fostered by these cumulative moments, which progressively change the energy and perspective.

This procedure also involves routines. Creating a consistent fitness routine fosters dedication and facilitates incorporating activity into everyday life. Finding a workout partner may increase motivation because of the companionship and shared experiences, which turn a routine that could otherwise seem like a drudgery into something fun. Laughter and support work together to form the experience's binding agent.

STARTING IS OFTEN THE most difficult part. Concentrating on the purpose of activity might be beneficial on days when motivation seems elusive. Making an intention changes the viewpoint from one of duty to one of opportunity, whether the goal is to reduce stress, increase vitality, or just enjoy the present. A attitude that promotes wellbeing is fostered by seeing activity as a gift to oneself.

Exercise's social component provides further advantages for those suffering from persistent depression. A feeling of community is fostered by group courses, which serve as a reminder that people have comparable challenges and victories. This group spirit has the potential to spread, turning lonely exercises into vibrant events full of encouragement and support.

Mindfulness permeates the exercise as movement becomes second nature. One develops a stronger connection with themselves when they pay attention to how their body feels during exercise, whether it's the burn of exercising muscles or the release of stress. This knowledge fosters emotional resilience in addition to improving physical performance.

TRYING OUT NEW THINGS provides a fun factor that makes you want to exercise more. Variety and excitement may be added by taking a few different fitness courses, joining a local hiking club, or trying out a new activity. By encouraging a spirit of adventure, this attitude of discovery transforms exercise from a duty into a joyful experience.

There are many ways in which movement and mental health are related. Exercise has been shown to improve mood and cognitive performance time and time again. Frequent exercise acts as a natural cure for the weight that often accompanies anxiety and sadness by reducing its symptoms.

Additionally, exercise is a really effective way to process emotions. Physical exercise may provide a safe way to express emotions that might otherwise seem too much to handle. The body offers a conduit for emotional release, promoting recovery and development, whether it is via a calming yoga flow, a strenuous exercise, or a cathartic run.

IN THIS COMPLEX DANCE, movement and nutrition are also intertwined. Eating the correct nutrients gives the body the energy it needs to workout. A nutrient-rich, well-balanced diet improves both cognitive and physical performance, fostering a positive relationship between one's emotions and food intake. The idea that taking care of the body promotes improved mental clarity and emotional stability is supported by this interconnection.

Embracing moderate movement might provide comfort during times of overload. When the world seems too heavy, exercises like stretching, strolling, or even gentle yoga may be a haven. They reinforce the concept that every stride forward matters by reminding people that even little acts of movement have enormous power.

DURING THIS JOURNEY, listening to the body becomes a crucial skill. A caring connection with oneself is fostered by being aware of and respecting one's own boundaries. Burnout may result from overexertion, yet moderate exercise benefits the body and mind and fosters a long-term, sustainable habit.

The cumulative benefits of regular activity become apparent as the days go by. Exercise, which was previously a difficult activity, becomes a beloved habit. Progress is seen in resilience, emotional stability, mental clarity, and physical strength. Every session turns into a celebration of success, strengthening the link between the mind and body.

Remembering the power of movement acts as a reminder at times of uncertainty or difficulty. Every decision, no matter how little, adds to a greater story of recovery and development. Every person's journey is different, with movement serving as a catalyst and paving the path to freedom from the voices that lurk in the background.

A route to regaining happiness and purpose is provided by this investigation of exercise and mental health. People are encouraged to live life to the fullest, gaining power in each stride, breath, and moment spent with others. One might cultivate a deep metamorphosis by just moving their body, negotiating life's challenges with poise and fortitude.

CHAPTER 5
BUILDING MEANINGFUL CONNECTIONS AND SUPPORT SYSTEMS

MAKING RELATIONSHIPS with other people may change the healing process and provide a strong support system during trying times. As relationships develop, the loneliness that often accompanies persistent depression disappears, creating an atmosphere that allows vulnerability to thrive. Genuine connections turn into a haven where people may talk about their challenges and rejoice in their successes.

Interaction with people brings warmth into the chilly times of life. A kind wave from a neighbor, a fortuitous meeting at a coffee shop, or a mutual interest in a pastime may all serve as the catalyst for the beginning of a friendship. Every encounter sows the seeds of connection, fostering the long-term development of connections. It requires readiness to welcome such times, accept invitations, and seek out company when it is most convenient to isolate oneself.

VULNERABILITY IS IMPORTANT in these linkages. People may freely share their opinions and emotions in an intimate setting created by sharing experiences. The emotional burden is lessened by this exchange, which may be like taking off a bulky garment on a warm day. Authenticity is promoted when someone listens without passing judgment, telling others that their difficulties are real and acknowledged.

Through these connections, support networks develop, providing not just company but also direction and motivation. In times of need, reaching out to friends or family allows for empathy and compassion. These intimate moments, whether they take the form of a heartfelt discussion or a straightforward text message, serve as a reminder that people are not alone in their experiences.

THIS FEELING OF BELONGING may be strengthened by taking part in group activities. Opportunities to meet others with similar interests might be found via classes, organizations, or community gatherings. Participating in group activities, such as a hiking club or reading club, promotes a feeling of togetherness. Strangers become friends as a result of conversations that spontaneously arise around common interests.

Additionally, digital channels facilitate connections. People may encourage one another and share their tales via virtual gatherings, social media groups, and online forums. Initial hesitancy may be reduced by the anonymity of the internet, which makes it simpler to express emotions without the pressure of instantaneous presence. Sincere friendships may thrive despite geographical distance when this connection develops into deeper partnerships.

Creating a network of support goes beyond friendships. Healing may be greatly aided by professional relationships. Support groups, therapists, and counselors provide individualized direction and encouragement. Speaking with mental health specialists may lead to new coping mechanisms, resilience building, and a better understanding of the intricacies of depression. As people learn to trust in the healing process, these connections provide a foundation for personal development.

FEELINGS OF CONNECTEDNESS may be strengthened via community participation. A feeling of purpose may be developed by volunteering for nearby nonprofits, taking part in community activities, or joining advocacy organizations. One develops a stronger bond with the community when they contribute to something greater than themselves. Individuals are brought together by these common objectives, which prioritize the welfare of the group.

Giving brings satisfaction and lessens feelings of loneliness, changing one's connection with oneself and others.

In these exchanges, self-awareness blossoms. Establishing appropriate limits in partnerships is facilitated by an understanding of individual needs. Emotional well-being is fostered by knowing when to participate and when to withdraw. It's crucial to be around by encouraging people who provide rather than take away from one's vitality. This discernment creates a network that fosters development and makes room for a supportive and upbeat atmosphere.

In these interactions, trust develops over time, strengthening ties. Being open and vulnerable with people creates a comfortable environment and opens the door to more meaningful relationships. Honest discussions where people may share their hopes and anxieties are made possible by trust. By serving as a reminder to all parties involved that vulnerability is a strength rather than a weakness, these open moments foster empathy.

IT MIGHT BE INTIMIDATING to navigate the intricacies of establishing relationships. It takes bravery to get over shyness or rejection anxiety. However, the benefits of venturing beyond of one's comfort zone often surpass the initial pain. Little actions like striking up a discussion or joining a group might result in deep connections that enhance life's path.

Developing thankfulness strengthens these bonds. A greater appreciation for the assistance received is fostered by acknowledging the importance of connections. Thanking loved ones, friends, or coworkers improves the relationships formed. Small tokens of gratitude or a sincere "thank you" are examples of simple gestures that strengthen good dynamics in relationships.

It takes work and intention to keep these relationships going. Frequent check-ins, whether by phone calls, messaging, or in-person encounters, foster the connections that have been built. Providing updates on life's highs and lows strengthens the support system. others are reminded that they are surrounded by others who really care by these encounters, which turn become lifelines.

Connections gain depth when the idea of reciprocity is embraced. Supporting one another in return strengthens the relationship. A feeling of equilibrium is promoted by hearing about the hardships of others or by acknowledging their successes. This reciprocal interaction strengthens the healing process for all parties involved by fostering a thriving network where everyone feels appreciated.

RELATIONSHIPS BECOME sources of inspiration as they develop. Friends who support personal development and self-compassion act as change agents. Discussions about objectives, hopes, and dreams might inspire people to follow their interests, which may have been neglected due to depression. Everyone is reminded of the strength of connection by this common trip, which turns into a source of optimism.

Healing happens organically as a result of these meaningful interactions. Resilience is fostered by emotional support, shared experiences, and group development, which makes it easier for people to deal with the challenges of depression. These connections give ordinary situations vitality and elevate them from ordinary to remarkable.

EVERY RELATIONSHIP adds a thread to the tapestry of life, weaving it together with empathy, understanding, and support. The path to recovery turns into a communal experience that is full of growth, sorrow, and laughter. The sound of self-doubt subsides as ties become stronger, giving way to a chorus of heartfelt support.

In the end, the process of establishing relationships changes the mental health landscape. A journey that may begin as a lonely one develops into a thriving community where people support and flourish alongside one another. Everyone is reminded that they are never really alone by the way friendship and support work together to create a space where healing is not only possible but also celebrated.

Recognizing the Power of Community

Every contact carries the pulse of community, echoing with a communal energy that can boost even the lowest of moods. People find strength in getting together, sharing experiences, and creating relationships that go beyond the norm. Every interaction has the capacity to produce a tapestry made from common experiences, offering a chance to feel understanding and solidarity.

THERE ARE MANY OTHER ways that communities may be formed, including via local organizations, interest groups, internet forums, and neighborhoods. Every location turns into a haven, welcoming those looking for understanding and company. In these settings, individuals meet others who travel comparable routes, and common hardships foster an atmosphere full of compassion. People may overcome the loneliness that often accompanies mental health issues when they realize that others are fighting similar struggles.

When you go into a communal environment, you could feel nervous, but the kind smiles might make you feel better. Stories of success and adversity are carried by conversations that flow like rivers. Every voice emphasizes how each person's journey adds to the overall story, adding a note to the symphony of our common humanity. Leaning in, listening, and sharing one's truth are all encouraged when one realizes that these places are there to support one another.

RESILIENCE IS FOSTERED by community involvement. Shared interests, such as volunteer work, reading clubs, or group exercise, naturally lead to the development of relationships. These activities evolve into chances for development and healing rather than only being get-togethers. Together, people commemorate life events, support one another through adversity, and build a network that promotes mental health and wellbeing.

Community may be a lifeline during times of sorrow. Even the worst days may be brightened by a kind smile or a word of encouragement, reminding them that there is always hope. Someone who is feeling lost might be greatly impacted by the simple act of asking how their neighbor is doing or offering to help. These actions may not seem like much, yet they have a big impact and encourage people to be kind, understanding, and compassionate.

Communities flourish because of their variety, which is a source of great strength. People may learn from each other because of the many origins, experiences, and viewpoints that make up the colorful tapestry. Everyone's horizons are expanded via the development that is fostered by the mixing of cultures, ideas, and thinking. Being exposed to other points of view encourages introspection and fosters a greater comprehension of the human condition.

GIVING BACK STRENGTHENS the bond between people. People engage in a reciprocal loop that fosters a sense of community when they donate their time or skills. One might develop a feeling of purpose by mentoring others, planning events, or volunteering for neighborhood charity. People are motivated to connect and share their talents with people around them by this purpose, which arouses passion and excitement. People get a stronger sense of belonging when they see the results of their labors.

In communities, gratitude becomes a powerful force. Recognizing other people's work creates a positive and appreciative atmosphere. Bonds are strengthened when you acknowledge when someone goes above and beyond, whether it's by listening or offering assistance. Celebrating these occasions with small gestures, such as a shout-out at a gathering or a sincere thank-you, strengthens the group's resolve to support one another.

KEEPING AN OPEN MIND and heart is essential to creating lasting interactions. Being vulnerable while interacting with people might be intimidating. Sharing personal hardships, however, fosters closer relationships and dismantles the walls that isolation often creates. Real discussions take place, resulting in fresh insights and relationships that are sincere and life-changing.

The idea of mutual help thrives in communal contexts. A strong feeling of security is produced when you realize that there are others standing by your side, willing to listen or provide a helping hand. People no longer feel like they are fighting their inner demons alone. Rather, they join a wider movement, a group of people working together to find healing and development. This relationship builds resilience, laying the groundwork for both individual and group development.

People unintentionally nourish themselves as they nurture their societies. Interacting with others who have gone through similar things to you serves to emphasize how important connections are. People who talk about their difficulties often find that resilience is bred by vulnerability. By expressing one's truth, one encourages others to do the same, creating a cycle of transparency that fortifies the community's bonds.

Spending time in public areas provides opportunities for celebration and happiness. Long-lasting memories are created by the simple joy of a shared meal, the thrill of organizing a neighborhood event, or the laughing over a cup of coffee. These encounters enhance lives by transforming transient relationships into enduring ones.

Being a member of a community makes you realize that no one's path is defined by the difficulties they face in life. Rather, they turn into common experiences that unite people. Every individual's tale reminds everyone that they are part of something bigger and gives the community narrative depth and complexity.

Exploration is encouraged by the power that comes from community. People may experiment with various hobbies, adopt new roles, and discover the many dimensions of who they are. Entering a supportive setting enables exploration without worrying about criticism. Whether it's sharing artistic creations, talking about personal challenges, or acting in a local theater, these activities turn into a celebration of bravery and development.

PEOPLE ENCOURAGE ONE another to seek personal development as their connections get stronger. New ideas are generated via conversations, which result in a common path of introspection and investigation. When someone starts a new project, the community comes together to support and encourage them. This support inspires people to pursue their goals and follow their interests, reminding them that they have the ability to make a difference in their own life.

Beyond the person, the strength of community has far-reaching effects. People outside the organization may be inspired by the tales told in these areas, attracting new members who might benefit from the group's assistance. Every additional participant broadens the circle of empathy and understanding while enhancing the story.

A DEDICATION TO INCLUSION is also necessary for fostering community. Deeper relationships are made possible by acknowledging the need for safe environments where everyone is accepted. Everyone can make a significant contribution to the community if there is an open discussion that values different points of view. In the end, this inclusion strengthens the group by boosting discussions and experiences.

In the end, change is invited when one embraces the power of community. It enables people to overcome their situations, building resilience that may result in significant recovery. Each bond created becomes a thread in the greater fabric of life, which is then interwoven to generate a stunning depiction of our common humanity. People may get the help they need via community, which serves as a reminder that they are all a part of something much bigger than themselves.

Asking for Help Without Fear

Asking for assistance can frequently feel like negotiating a maze, a labyrinth of hesitation and anxiety. A thousand ideas fly through the head, all of them centered on the dread of being vulnerable. What are they going to think? Are they going to pass judgment? Or worse, will they turn away when they see the holes in one's armor? However, overcoming that barrier of doubt allows for deep healing and a sense of community.

A lonely suffering may become a shared experience just by reaching out. It's about acknowledging the burden one has and realizing that there are those who can lessen it. Talking to someone, whether it a friend, relative, or therapist, starts a process that transforms a personal struggle into a group struggle. Speaking out creates a supportive environment where people may find comfort in knowing one another.

EMOTIONS SPIKE WHEN you picture that initial action, like picking up the phone or sending that SMS. Fear and excitement combine to create a powerful combination that can immobilize. Ideas bounce around: "What if they don't answer?or "What happens if they don't comprehend?However, there is a ton of promise in that instant. Every voice raised, every communication delivered, has the possibility of a connection. With the comfort of an open ear, the dread that lurks like a shadow might vanish.

Uncertainty may start the discussion, but authenticity comes from being vulnerable. Even in the most basic terms, expressing emotions builds a bond. "I need someone to talk to" or "I've been feeling down" are examples of invitations. These kinds of remarks help to break the ice and turn difficult situations into candid conversations. The weight suddenly seems lighter as empathy replaces loneliness and understanding enters the room.

DEVELOPING THIS RELATIONSHIP via dialogue promotes a feeling of belonging. Each person has a unique story of hardship and success. Others are often inspired to share their own experiences when someone else opens up. Everyone contributes to the fabric of our common humanity that is created by this interaction. By speaking out, people draw others into the discussion and start a chain reaction that promotes group healing.

In these conversations, language is important. Careful word choice may promote open communication and establish a comfortable environment. There is more space for discussion when ideas are framed as individual experiences rather than absolute facts. Saying "I feel overwhelmed" instead of "You don't understand" turns the discussion from a conflict into a cooperative investigation. This little change makes room for empathy, which improves the effectiveness and supportiveness of the exchange.

SOCIAL STIGMAS ARE often associated with seeking assistance, especially when it comes to mental health. Stereotypes wait in the dark to deter those who are in need. Vulnerability is often mistaken for weakness, however accepting one's challenges is a sign of strength. Recognizing that everyone has challenges fosters a common understanding that goes beyond stigma. Being brave enough to show one's feelings may spark change for both the person and the society at large.

Knowing that the appropriate support is available is essential to navigating the process of seeking assistance. Finding people who really listen, affirm, and support you may have a profound impact. Although friends and family are often willing to give assistance, experts like therapists or counselors may provide further resources and techniques. Their knowledge may help people adopt better coping strategies and cognitive processes, which will promote healing even more.

Reaching out may often seem like an empowering exercise. It turns hopeless sentiments into proactive measures for healing. Every time someone speaks out, they take back a piece of who they are. The more people seek for assistance, the more instinctive it gets. A positive feedback loop that emphasizes the value of community support is created by this repetition, which cultivates an openness-promoting habit.

THIS TECHNIQUE TAKES on a new level when done in group settings. Community gatherings, seminars, and support groups provide forums for people dealing with comparable issues to exchange experiences. People may see firsthand the power of shared vulnerability in these settings, where the group energy fosters healing. These events provide comfort as well as coping mechanisms for dealing with the intricacies of mental health.

In many situations, listening is just as important as speaking. It may change you to hear other people's tales. One's personal experience is often reflected in the stories recounted, fostering empathy and unity. This conversation strengthens the idea that people are never really alone by fostering a feeling of belonging. Creating relationships based on common experiences might encourage individuals to keep reaching out and build resilience.

Recognizing the possibility of rejection is another aspect of comprehending the emotional terrain of seeking assistance. It's OK that not every approach will get an understanding answer. Every event has important lessons to offer. While some interactions will lead to new opportunities, some may not. Acknowledging this fact enables people to persevere in their pursuit of connection without taking failures personally.

It takes time to establish a network of support. It takes time for relationships to develop. It takes work, patience, and care to plant the seeds of connection. The process entails contacting many people and looking at various assistance systems. Regardless of its effectiveness, every encounter advances our knowledge of the many ways people might connect.

THE COMMUNITY IS STRENGTHENED when a culture of transparency around mental health issues is established. People encourage others to be vulnerable and real by setting an example. This group change has the power to change attitudes and turn stigma into understanding. As the discussion deepens, people are inspired to ask for assistance fearlessly.

Every attempt to communicate, whether by text, phone, or in-person meeting, contributes to a greater healing movement. Every voice adds to the story of our common humanity and serves as a reminder that people are not defined by their difficulties. Rather, they function as hubs, creating a support system that endures even the most trying circumstances.

In the end, asking for assistance develops into a continuous conversation that is full of possibilities and promise. Every discussion builds on the one before it, resulting in an ongoing stream of comprehension and assistance. In addition to helping people, this connection journey enhances communities by creating links that withstand the ups and downs of life's obstacles.

When people accept their voices and realize they have the ability to ask for help and build relationships, empowerment blooms. Despite the challenges along the way, every step made to seek assistance turns fear into strength. Reaching out turns into a powerful statement, reminding people that all voices count and that they may work together to build a healing symphony.

CHAPTER 6
MINDFULNESS, MEDITATION, AND ALTERNATIVE THERAPIES

IN THE MIDST OF THE stress of everyday life, mindfulness and meditation can seem like distant disciplines that are just out of grasp. However, when accepted, they provide avenues for clarity and serenity that may change what it's like to live with chronic depression. These techniques provide a soft anchor in the whirlpool of ideas and feelings, bringing people back to the here and now and encouraging internal healing.

Imagine sitting comfortably, closing your eyes, and breathing in and out with ease. Every breath serves as a subtle reminder to stay alive and to get back in touch with oneself. Thoughts flood in, racing and overlapping, yet there's a need to watch them objectively. This little gesture fosters awareness by enabling one to take a step back and see emotions as fleeting phenomena rather than permanent installations. As time passes, it becomes clear that the present is more important than the responsibilities of the past.

MINDFULNESS HAS THE power to elevate routine tasks into meaningful encounters. Imagine doing the dishes as the warm water swirls over your hands and the aromas of soap mix with the surrounding air. There is a chance to be present when you give this work your whole attention, experiencing the textures and hearing the noises. When done intentionally, every task turns into a daily routine that fosters mindfulness and thankfulness, a kind of meditation.

Meditation provides a haven, a secure environment where ideas can flow and the mind can roam. There are other methods, such as body scans, loving-kindness, or concentrated attention, each offering a different path for investigation. While some people enjoy the simplicity of quiet thought, others may find comfort in guided sessions. The secret is to discover what speaks to you and let the practice develop naturally.

Expectations often surface as the voyage progresses, pulling at the mind like a kid vying for attention. Frustration might result from the desire to attain a perfect state of serenity overshadowing the experience. But it's important to keep in mind that acceptance is what meditation feeds on. While some days may cause unrest, others may seem easy. A greater awareness of oneself and resilience are fostered by accepting this ebb and flow.

Even the most basic actions become chances for personal development when mindfulness is included into everyday routines. Walking becomes into a dance with the ground, where one grounds themselves in the present moment with each mindful stride. A meal becomes a sensory experience as the tastes and sensations come to life. People nurture their souls as well as their bodies by relishing every mouthful.

For those negotiating the intricacies of depression, mindfulness is a powerful ally. According to research, consistent practice may lessen symptoms while fostering resilience and mental health. The beauty concealed in every moment is revealed when the mind, which is often entangled in negativity, starts to untangle. Healing is facilitated by a mindful approach that promotes a change from self-criticism to self-compassion.

Apart from mindfulness and meditation, alternative treatments can prove to be beneficial allies throughout the healing process. Movement-based exercises like yoga, tai chi, and others combine mindfulness with physical activity to foster a healthy body-mind connection. Yoga positions encourage awareness and encourage people to respect their bodies and their limits. A feeling of connection and grounding is facilitated by the soft stretching and breathing pattern.

ANOTHER IMPORTANT FACTOR in this healing process is nature. Being outside in the fresh air and among trees helps people rediscover something bigger than themselves. Nature is a salve that calms the mind and uplifts the soul. Hiking, gardening, or just lounging in a park may all be considered meditation exercises that let people lose themselves in the sights and sounds of nature. A symphony of rustling leaves, chirping birds, and a light wind fosters wellbeing.

Investigating artistic endeavors gives the healing process a new depth. Writing, music, and art all provide ways to express and let go of oneself. By letting emotions freely flow into the painting, paper, or music, these techniques function as a kind of meditation. Creativity has a profoundly positive impact on the soul and cultivates feelings of pleasure and success. Doodling, even in its most basic form, may provide an escape, a chance to access the subconscious and uncover emotions that are concealed.

Supplements and herbal treatments have gained popularity as supplemental methods for mental wellness. They may enhance general well-being but cannot replace expert medical care. Adaptogens, like rhodiola or ashwagandha, have received attention for their capacity to lower stress and increase resilience. Including these organic components in one's daily routine promotes a comprehensive strategy that takes into account one's body, mind, and soul.

Adopting alternative treatments empowers people and enables them to actively participate in their own recovery process. Every technique, whether it yoga, mindfulness, or artistic expression, serves as a tool in one's own toolbox. By trying out different strategies, people might find what works and create a special support system.

A CRUCIAL COMPONENT of this journey is still connection. A feeling of belonging is fostered by sharing experiences with others, whether via friendships or support groups. Talking about alternative treatments and mindfulness builds a network of knowledge. People may support one another in times of need and inspire one another by exchanging effective strategies.

When there is purpose and goal, the path through persistent depression seems less overwhelming. One moment at a time, people may take back their life by adopting mindfulness, meditation, and alternative treatments. The struggle is turned into a chance for development and learning as each little step leads to a closer relationship with oneself and the outside environment.

It takes time to find the ideal balance between these techniques. It will feel heavier on certain days and lighter on others. Every event adds to the general fabric of life, which is made up of strands of fortitude and resiliency. By taking an open approach to healing, people create a space that is conducive to change, which enables the layers of depression to come off.

Ultimately, the process of healing with mindfulness, meditation, and complementary treatments develops in stages, each of which offers fresh perspectives and chances for development. People learn to embrace life's ups and downs and trust their gut feelings as they travel this path. Being present becomes a powerful discipline that serves as a reminder that there is always hope for recovery and rejuvenation. Investigating these methods gives people the means to create a better, more satisfying future in addition to a means of escaping the chaos.

The Benefits of Mindfulness in Daily Life

In today's hectic world, mindfulness seems as a mild cure, a means of keeping oneself rooted in the here and now. The simplicity of mindfulness is its core; it provides a means of completely embracing each moment, transforming ordinary situations into chances for development and interpersonal relationships.

IMAGINE GOING OUTDOORS and experiencing the warmth of the sun against the chilly morning air. Every breath turns into a deliberate action that draws in the surroundings. During these times, the cacophony subsides, the mental chatter stops, and clarity emerges. It's about enjoying the richness of the present moment and paying attention to the little things that are sometimes overlooked.

By integrating mindfulness into everyday activities, regular chores become meaningful rituals. Imagine the experience of sipping a cup of tea. One may take the time to enjoy the scent and the warmth of the cup in hand rather than blindly consuming coffee while browsing through a phone. Grounding oneself in the moment rather than rushing to the next commitment, each sip turns into a little celebration of the senses. Spending every minute to the fullest enhances life and fosters a greater feeling of gratitude.

Being attentive serves as a buffer against the constant onslaught of stimuli that life presents. Because stress is so weighty, it may slip into the body and mind, impairing judgment and fostering negativity. However, mindfulness teaches people to identify stressors before they become more severe. A more measured reaction is made possible by the simple act of stopping, taking a deep breath, and examining sensations objectively. This knowledge changes how people behave, enabling them to make decisions instead of just reacting to events.

Under the impact of mindfulness, interpersonal interactions often blossom. People have deeper interactions and stronger bonds with friends, family, and coworkers when they practice being present. Imagine conversing with a buddy while seated across from them, not only waiting for your time to speak but really paying attention. Relationships may flourish in honesty because of the connection and understanding this presence cultivates. The depth of connection fills the void left by distractions, forming a network of support that benefits both sides.

THE ADVANTAGES OF MINDFULNESS also extend to emotional health. People who suffer from persistent depression often have a propensity to ruminate—to continuously cycle through unpleasant ideas. However, by practicing mindfulness, people might see these thinking patterns as fleeting clouds in a wide sky rather than as truths. The power that ideas contain may be gently released by seeing them without attachment. This change may loosen the hold of hopelessness and provide room for more optimistic emotions to surface.

Practicing mindfulness increases one's capacity for self-compassion. Life may be a tough critic, with harsh and judgmental inner monologues. This story may be changed by engaging in mindfulness practices. The severity of self-criticism starts to lessen when people are patient and compassionate to themselves. This self-care fosters an atmosphere that is conducive to recovery. People become resilient against the obstacles life presents by accepting their flaws and showing compassion.

Being mindful can be incorporated easily into everyday life and is not only for peaceful times spent on a meditation cushion. Walking's cadence offers a chance to practice mindfulness. The body may grow more connected to the ground with each intentional step. Observing the sensations of feet on the floor, breathing patterns, and arm movements results in a smooth dance with life. Movement turns into a kind of meditation that energizes the spirit and grounds people in the here and now.

Practicing mindfulness every day promotes innovation and creativity. There are more opportunities for new thoughts and solutions to surface when the mind is free of distractions. Letting rid of inflexible mental patterns encourages spontaneity and motivates people to go into new areas of their life. A mindful mentality encourages the capacity to think creatively, whether one is brainstorming in a professional context or tackling personal obstacles.

A GREAT SETTING FOR practicing mindfulness is often found in nature. People are invited to fully appreciate the beauty of the earth as they stroll through a park with trees, birds, and the gentle rustling of leaves all around them. The exercise is improved by the vivid colors and noises, which constitute an essential component of the experience. A feeling of belonging that promotes mental wellbeing is fostered by nature, which serves as a subtle reminder of how intertwined everything is.

Perspective is a gift of mindfulness. Focusing on the here and now helps people to enjoy the short times in life. The tenderness of a loved one's touch, the flavor of a beloved meal, or a child's soothing giggle may all be treasured. This appreciation invites thankfulness into daily life by changing the emphasis from what is missing to what is plentiful.

People who practice mindfulness may discover that their physical health improves as well. According to research, practicing mindfulness may boost immunity, reduce blood pressure, and enhance sleep quality. The body and mind dance delicately together, and when one does well, the other usually does too. People who practice mindfulness are better able to pay attention to their body and know when to take breaks or partake in nutritious activities.

THE BENEFITS OF MINDFULNESS practice may be increased when done in a group setting. Participating in community courses or mindfulness circles fosters a shared environment for learning and development. The practice is improved by the energy of group practice, which promotes support and accountability. This kind of interaction with others helps people feel like they belong and serves as a reminder that they are not traveling alone.

Additionally, journaling may be an effective mindfulness technique. By putting pen to paper, one may process feelings and ideas and produce a physical record of events. People may see patterns in their thoughts and actions by engaging in this activity, which encourages introspection and understanding. Journaling allows people to examine difficulties, celebrate victories, and get a deeper knowledge of who they are.

Mindfulness acts as an anchor and a stabilizing factor during times of intense emotion. Acknowledging emotions without passing judgment makes it easier for people to deal with life's highs and lows. They may see anger, sorrow, and worry as passing feelings rather of letting them consume them. This method develops emotional intelligence by enabling people to react intelligently rather than impulsively.

Practicing mindfulness may even increase output. The quality of work often increases when the mind learns to concentrate on a single activity at a time. In our fast-paced society, multitasking is sometimes seen as a badge of pride, yet it may also result in fatigue and lower productivity. Adopting single-tasking allows people to experience the fulfillment that comes from purposefully and thoughtfully finishing activities.

A CHANGE IN PERSPECTIVE is encouraged by mindfulness, which pushes people to welcome life's path with curiosity and openness. The process, the little moments that weave life together, is what's beautiful. Mindfulness serves as a beacon of light, shedding light on the way to recovery and rejuvenation as people learn to negotiate the intricacies of their experiences.

Life emerges in vivid hues when mindfulness is practiced, a tapestry woven with peaceful, self-discovering, and connecting moments. People start to change their tales from ones of despair to ones of promise and hope by developing this skill. Every thought and breath turns into a step on the path to a fuller, more satisfying life.

Exploring Complementary Therapies

The investigation of complementary treatments stands out as a ray of hope for individuals negotiating the intricacies of emotional discomfort in the constantly changing field of mental health. These strategies often blend in well with conventional techniques, providing a comprehensive viewpoint that respects the complexity of the human experience. People may find recovery routes that suit their own requirements by adopting these methods.

IMAGINE ENTERING A space that is filled with soothing aromas and gentle light, where the air is heavy with the promise of recovery. With its combination of essential oils, aromatherapy encourages people to undergo significant changes in their mood and mental clarity. The aromas of citrus or lavender swirl in the air, enveloping the mind like a cozy hug and releasing the victim from the grip of worry. Just breathing in these scents promotes relaxation, improves wellbeing, and creates a peaceful environment for introspection.

Complementary treatments are more successful when mindfulness is included into them. Imagine an aromatherapy-enhanced guided meditation where calming voices softly lead thoughts inward as the fragrance of chamomile permeates the air. This combination promotes a feeling of calm in the midst of turmoil by encouraging deeper connections with oneself. People may tap their inner resources and find strength by participating in these periods of silence. By practicing mindfulness, the cacophony of the outer world subsides, exposing the inner silence.

Through movement and breathing, yoga integrates the body and mind, and it often emerges as a potent alternative treatment. People develop awareness of their bodily presence as they go through positions, meaningfully reestablishing a connection with their bodies. Each movement is guided by the breath's rhythm, resulting in a dance that relieves tension and increases strength and flexibility. Yoga's transformational qualities foster mental and physical fortitude, reminding practitioners that they have the means to overcome obstacles in life.

THE MIND-BODY LINK becomes more important when persistent emotional suffering is present. By treating the physical symptoms of stress and anxiety, complementary treatments such as massage therapy and acupuncture provide pathways to recovery. Imagine the soft prick of needles put in key locations to open energy channels and release bottled-up emotions. As the body regains its natural flow, this exercise promotes a feeling of balance and strengthens the link between physical and emotional well-being.

Furthermore, investigating nutritional techniques demonstrates the significant influence that food may have on brain clarity and mood. A diet high in whole foods, omega-3 fatty acids, and antioxidants is often recommended by nutritionists. Imagine a dish full with bright fruits, veggies, seeds, and nuts. These meals provide vital nutrients that promote brain health, balancing mood and improving cognitive abilities. By realizing that their diet has a significant impact on their general health, people may gain control over their lives.

In the field of complementary treatments, herbal medicines are also quite important. Those looking for natural help have several alternatives thanks to the ancient understanding of herbal medicine. Think about the mood-boosting benefits of St. John's Wort or the relaxing qualities of valerian root. People who include these herbs into their everyday routines often discover that they are better able to manage mood swings. People are encouraged to investigate the advantages of plants as friends in their path to balance because nature offers a huge pharmacy of therapeutic resources.

ANOTHER WAY TO EXPLORE is via art therapy, which enables people to communicate feelings that may otherwise go unsaid. Painting, sketching, or creating are examples of creative pursuits that provide a release by turning emotions into material forms. This activity promotes self-expression and offers a secure environment free from linguistic limitations to examine difficult feelings.

Through art, people uncover new facets of themselves and gain understanding that may lead to more profound healing.

In a similar vein, music therapy opens up a channel for emotional inquiry by using the therapeutic potential of sound. Through active engagement or passive listening, music evokes emotions that are often hidden under the surface. Think about the ability of a well-known tune to instantly elicit memories or change feelings. People are encouraged to engage with their emotions via music therapy, which facilitates a cathartic release that often results in significant discoveries and change.

The advantages of individual practices may be increased by participating in community-based complementary treatments. Group courses, seminars, and support groups provide chances for interaction and experience sharing. Imagine taking part in yoga classes or guided mindfulness exercises while sitting in a circle with others who have comparable challenges. People are reminded that they are not traveling alone by this communal energy, which cultivates a feeling of belonging. Healing may occur in a supportive setting because to the common knowledge and experiences that are shared in these settings, which often promote personal development.

A proactive approach to mental health is promoted by incorporating alternative treatments into everyday life. By developing a self-care program that incorporates many modalities, people may take control of their health. This schedule may include yoga to invigorate the body, meditation in the morning, a hearty meal full of good fats, and a stroll in the evening to relax. Every component works as a thread to weave self-care into a tapestry that supports the body and the mind.

The efficacy of these treatments is significantly influenced by the power of intention. People encourage opportunities for change when they approach their healing process with inquiry and openness. Establishing goals, whether they be to embrace pleasure, relieve stress, or foster tranquility, provides a path to recovery. Every practice turns becomes a chance to be in line with these goals, giving everyday life direction and significance.

Complementary treatments often encourage people to accept their particular healing journeys. Every trip is unique, therefore there is no one-size-fits-all strategy. Part of the inquiry involves trying out different modalities to see what resonates. Being open to trying new things might lead to surprising discoveries and reveal avenues that could have stayed undiscovered.

IN THE END, INVESTIGATING alternative treatments promotes a better comprehension of oneself. People discover the knowledge that exists within them when they learn to listen to their bodies and emotions via various disciplines. By cultivating self-compassion, this understanding makes it possible to navigate obstacles more gently. As people accept their potential for development and healing, the journey turns into a dance, a smooth transition between practices and insights.

People may develop a feeling of empowerment and agency by embracing alternative treatments. They reclaim their stories by actively participating in their well-being, crafting tales of resiliency and optimism. The trip turns into a celebration of potential and a monument to the fortitude that comes from looking for other routes to recovery. People who investigate these options often find that they feel more connected to the world and themselves again, in addition to receiving relief from mental suffering.

SUMMARY

This manual serves as a lighthouse, shedding light on paths to recovery and self-discovery in a world sometimes overshadowed by the burden of persistent depression. Every page speaks to the hardships that many people go through, creating a tapestry of events that highlight the significant obstacles and unsung triumphs experienced on the path to emotional liberation. These chapters invite readers to set out on their own transformational journeys by combining personal tales with useful advice.

Investigating mental health takes center stage, revealing the sometimes misinterpreted intricacies of long-term depression. It transports readers to a realm where emotions flow like currents, sometimes tumultuous, at other times calm. This is not just a professional evaluation. Those who have experienced the loneliness of despair and the need for connection may relate to the words. It promotes an awareness that regaining control over one's own story begins with addressing one's emotions.

Throughout the book, several methods for escaping the grip of despair surface, each providing a distinct viewpoint on achieving liberation. Conversations on the importance of movement and fitness are interwoven with hands-on activities intended to foster mindfulness. The heart of the release that physical exercise may provide is encapsulated in imagery of limbs extending and brains clearing. Readers may feel themselves shedding the weight that hangs on too tightly with every drop of perspiration, turning their bodies into strong, resilient vessels.

THE STORY ESTABLISHES strong bonds, highlighting the value of community and support networks. Relationships may serve as lifelines at the most difficult times, as seen by the stories of friendship, empathy, and understanding that surface. By encouraging people to interact, the guide serves as a reminder that they are not alone. It depicts vulnerability, humor, and shared experiences as essential elements of recovery. As they recount their hardships and victories, readers may picture themselves seated in a circle with their voices blending together, forging an unbreakable tie of solidarity.

The tale illustrates the effectiveness of alternative therapy as the trip progresses. With a gentle twist, each chapter invites readers to delve further into the many techniques that provide solace and insight. The focus shifts to mindfulness practices, which help people focus on the here and now while letting their thoughts pass by like clouds. By teaching the technique of breathing possibilities and expelling stress, breathwork becomes a tool for anchoring. It is suggested that readers shut their eyes and sit quietly so that the rhythm of their breathing will cure them.

Creativity is explored as a powerful remedy for emotional suffering. Writing, music, and art all act as mediums for expressing emotions, letting them spill into paper or canvas. The manual emphasizes that creativity is more than perfection and encourages readers to take up a brush or pen. It's an encouragement to be untidy and to delve deeply into one's psyche without fear of criticism. Emotions transform into words, sounds, and colors in this hallowed place, allowing for self-expression and healing.

ANOTHER IMPORTANT ELEMENT that is woven into the fabric of healing is nutrition. The knowledge that what we eat affects our mental health is reflected in the emphasis on feeding the body. The book urges readers to develop a diet full of natural foods that are nutrient-dense and colorful. The recipes on these pages may inspire a love of cooking and transform meal preparation into a self-loving activity. The idea that every meal nourishes the body and the psyche is further supported by the way the perfume of spices and the sizzle of vegetables become symbols of metamorphosis.

The difficulties that come with asking for assistance are not downplayed in the book. It invites readers to question social norms by openly addressing the shame and fear often connected to mental health. The story is replete with calls to action, imploring readers to remove obstacles and ask for help without holding back. Readers are reminded that vulnerability is strength by the experiences of people who have traveled this path. Asking for assistance creates a feeling of community among those who have experienced similar difficulties by converting isolation into connection.

Readers see the human spirit's tenacity throughout the story. Every individual's tale reminds everyone that healing is a nonlinear process and offers a peek into the transformational power of hope. The book encourages readers to accept the complexity of their life by framing setbacks as chances for development rather than failures. This message strikes a deep chord with people, encouraging them to consider their particular journeys free from the weight of perfectionism.

The need of self-compassion is also emphasized throughout the book. It reminds readers that healing takes time and urges them to be nice to themselves. Techniques for developing self-love become crucial elements of the path. Moments of introspection and thankfulness turn into effective means of cultivating a positive outlook. In the process of turning self-doubt into a celebration of their individuality, readers may find themselves writing lists of qualities they like in themselves.

A FEELING OF EMPOWERMENT infuses the work as the latter chapters progress. It serves as a reminder to readers that they are in charge of their own recovery. Every tool that is offered serves as a stepping stone, inspiring people to bravely and intentionally construct their own pathways. The story ends with a call to accept life's intricacies and acknowledge that, despite the difficulties along the way, there are still many beautiful and meaningful moments.

This book serves as a monument to the human spirit's tenacity via its diverse range of experiences, wisdom, and helpful advice. It reminds readers that they are not alone in their challenges and promotes a feeling of understanding and belonging. The path to recovery turns into a communal experience, brimming with empathy, optimism, and the prospect of better times to come. Every page evokes the possibility of change, urging readers to take charge of their lives and take back control.

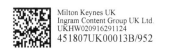
Milton Keynes UK
Ingram Content Group UK Ltd.
UKHW020916291124
451807UK00013B/952